Diabetes Educat

D1333698

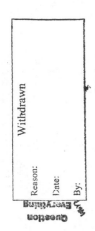

Education is not the filling of a pail but the lighting of a fire.
(W.B. Yeats 1865–1939)

Diabetes Education
Art, Science and Evidence

Edited by

Professor Trisha Dunning AM
RN, MEd, PhD, CDE, FRCNA
Chair in Nursing and Director Centre for Nursing and Allied Health Research
Deakin University and Barwon Health
Geelong, Victoria, Australia

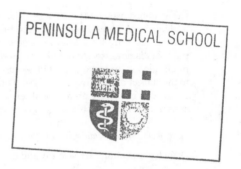

⊛WILEY-BLACKWELL
A John Wiley & Sons, Ltd., Publication

Library of Congress Cataloging-in-Publication Data

Diabetes education : art, science, and evidence / edited by Trisha Dunning.
     p. ; cm.
  Includes bibliographical references and index.
  ISBN 978-0-470-65605-1 (pbk. : alk. paper)
I. Dunning, Trisha.
[DNLM: 1. Diabetes Mellitus–therapy.   2. Diabetes Complications–prevention & control.   3. Patient Compliance.   4. Patient Education as Topic–methods.   5. Self Care.   WK 815]
  616.4′62–dc23
                                                    2012022778

A catalogue record for this book is available from the British Library.

Wiley also publishes its books in a variety of electronic formats. Some content that appears in print may not be available in electronic books.

Cover image: iLexx/iStockphoto
Cover design by Garth Stewart

Set in 9.5/12.5 pt Palatino by SPi Publisher Services, Pondicherry, India
Printed and bound in Malaysia by Vivar Printing Sdn Bhd

1   2013

Contents

List of Contributors

Jean-Phillippe Assal
President
Foundation for Research and Training
in Patient Education
Geneva, Switzerland

Tisiana Assal
Foundation for Research and Training
in Patient Education
Geneva, Switzerland

Trisha Dunning AM
Chair in Nursing and Director Centre
for Nursing and Allied Health Research
Deakin University
and
Barwon Health
Geelong, Victoria, Australia

Millie Glinsky
Indiana Regional Medical Center
Indiana, PA, USA

Kari Harno
LKT Dosentti FHIMSS
Kerava, Finland

Rhonda Lee
University of Pittsburgh Medical Center
Pittsburgh, PA, USA

Gretchen A. Piatt
Research Instructor
Division of Endocrinology and
Metabolism
School of Medicine
University of Pittsburgh
and
Director of Evaluation
Diabetes Institute
University of Pittsburgh
Pittsburgh, PA, USA

Michelle Robins
Nurse Practitioner
Corio Medical Centre
Corio, Victoria, Australia
and
Barwon Health
Geelong, Victoria, Australia

Norma Ryan
University of Pittsburgh Medical Center
Brownsville, PA, USA

Harsimran Singh
Department of Neurobehavioural Sciences
Behavioral Medicine Center
School of Medicine
University of Virginia
Charlottesville, VA, USA

Timothy Skinner
Director Rural Clinical School
University of Tasmania
Burnie, Tasmania, Australia

Jane Speight
The Australian Centre for Behavioural
Research in Diabetes
Diabetes Australia
Melbourne, Victoria, Australia
and
Centre for Mental Health and Well-being
Research
School of Psychology
Deakin University
Geelong, Victoria, Australia
and
AHP Research
Hornchurch, Essex, UK

Helen Thomasic
University of Pittsburgh Medical Center
Pittsburgh, PA, USA

Foreword

Trisha Dunning and her co-authors have compiled a book that knits state-of-the-art research findings with best clinical practice and good common sense to produce a most readable book of everyday application to clinicians and healthcare professionals in diabetes, as well as to the more enquiring person with diabetes seeking quality information. They are to be warmly congratulated for the many recommendations and helpful tips in the book, which derive from their lifetime in professional practice.

What particularly struck me was the vein of empathy with the person with diabetes that runs throughout the book. Those with diabetes so often fear that disappointing results at their clinic visit will earn disapproval or judgement, but the most welcome standpoint of the authors is to be non-judgemental and thoroughly supportive of those whom they serve, those with diabetes. For that reason, people starting their journey of diabetes and their carers would also profit from reading this book. Although learned, it contains a wealth of valuable information that can support them in the daily challenge of living with a chronic disease whose complications can, indeed, be life-threatening.

Although it is now over 25 years since I carried my comatose five-year-old daughter Kate into hospital with diabetic ketoacidosis, I shall never forget the sense of bewilderment and anxiety that engulfed me and the brutal realisation that this little child now faced a lifetime of insulin injections. How it would have helped to put everything in perspective for my wife, Naomi, and myself had we encountered at the outset, health practitioners of the sensitivity of the authors! That said, Kate was well cared for, and I can testify to the continuing gratitude parents and carers feel for those who care for their dependent child with diabetes. Together in Glasgow's Royal Hospital for Sick Children, a 'triangle of care' was formed between the caring professionals, my daughter Kate as the person with diabetes, and Naomi as the principal carer. When that triangle of care works well, there are immense benefits for all, and there are frequent references in the book to that potential for successful and mutually beneficial relationships between professionals and patients.

Without in any way denying the impressive support of the paediatric diabetologist, the key professional in that triangle of care was the Diabetes

Nurse Specialist. As unflappable as she was caring, she was indeed the educator, the source of advice, the encourager, the soother, the reassurer. She was the embodiment of all the fine attributes of the educator to which there is frequent implicit reference in the book. Without the ready access to such support, as carers we could easily have felt isolated and helpless when problems arose. It will come as no surprise that, to this day, I carry a standard for the nurse educator professionals.

This book is additionally welcome because not only does it summarise the best of diabetes care but it 'encourages educators to reflect on their philosophy of diabetes education and how they teach'. Educators are encouraged to excel and the myriad of practical recommendations—together with a vast anthology of references and research—should satisfy the most enquiring mind. Writing in my capacity as the incoming Global President of the International Diabetes Federation, I know instinctively that better informed, more accomplished educators will succeed in helping their patients to maintain better control of their diabetes.

It is not, however, just clinicians and healthcare professionals who can benefit from this book. As the information revolution advances inexorably, people with diabetes can inform themselves in a way that would have been unthinkable a generation ago. Kari Harno's compelling chapter on the Internet superhighway highlights the many exciting opportunities now opening up to harness technology to help those with diabetes to obtain optimal outcomes. It set me thinking of the many imaginative ways in which diabetes care and self-management could be revolutionised and improved. The 'quest for a better way', intrinsic in the human spirit, will bring undoubted benefits in the future to people with diabetes, reminding and supporting them to do the basic things that help maintain good control and a healthy life.

As a non-clinician, I found this book enjoyable to read but could not help relating the observations and anecdotes to the experiences of Kate, Naomi and myself in years past. I particularly liked Chapter 2 where Jane Speight and Harsimran Singh describe the journey of the person with diabetes and their observation that 'overcoming emotional reactions is likely to be one of the most important steps a person can take to manage their diabetes successfully. Yet, it is singularly the most overlooked aspect of diabetes care. Time and money are spent on screening for retinopathy and other complications of diabetes, and yet, very little effort is put into screening for emotional distress'. The authors of this chapter are right to highlight the imperative for health professionals to understand the role of the individual's family context in their diabetes management.

Reflecting honestly, I can see how daughter Kate's outcomes could have been improved if she had had access to proper psychosocial support at key times of her diabetes journey in adolescence and young adult life when leaving home weakened the parental influence on compliance. The importance of such psychosocial support is emphasised, directly and by implication, in many places in the book. I remain interested in the different ways in which such support can be offered and found myself in strong agreement with Gretchen Piatt's views on the beneficial effects of peer support. Whatever else, I am convinced that parents—hardwired to be protective—are not the best or right people to counsel when young people find compliance a tiresome burden, not least when they see their peers enjoying the diabetes-free existence they envy.

As with much else in life, effective communication can be the difference between success and failure. Trisha Dunning's chapter on effective communication is essential reading for those who daily interact with patients. Nowhere is there a greater requirement for effective communication than in the therapeutic patient education that she rightly identifies as an essential component of equipping the person with diabetes to achieve optimal outcomes. Trisha's chapters on education are pure gold, coupling practical experience with theory to produce guidance from which all health professionals can benefit. It is perhaps trite, but true, that continuing quality professional education is inseparable from good health outcomes, and without the benefits of good recurring education, the latter will be hard to achieve.

I hope that this book will be suggested if not prescribed reading for those who work in diabetes care. I hope too that those who read it, reflecting regularly as they do so, will find it relevant and useful and will thereby be empowered to care even more effectively for their patients with diabetes.

Sir Michael Hirst
June 2012

Preface

The word 'education' is interesting. It is derived from the Latin *educare*, to bring up, which is related to *educere*, to bring forth that which is within or bring out potential, and *ducere*, to lead. Significantly, *educare* also contains the word care.

There are many scientific books and papers about education including diabetes education—so why write another one? Ancient sages commanded 'physician know thyself' and suggested 'physician heal thyself'. Both these sentiments are at the heart of this book. At the end of each chapter is a list of questions to encourage educators to reflect on what they read and what they need to know to develop the courage to really teach, rather than just provide information.

Therein lies an important distinction—educators share their knowledge by providing information. The person who receives the information turns it into knowledge through complicated mental processes and is in control of what they learn and what they do with the information. Thus, an effective educator finds ways to develop the skills to 'sell' their messages by tailoring them to suit the individual. To do so, the educator must be open to new information sourced from numerous places and must know how to apply the information effectively. Above all, they need to actively cultivate the art of listening and being fully present in each encounter. Sometimes, just being there is enough.

Joslin emphasised the importance of diabetes education in the 1920s, but clear evidence for its value was not documented until the 1970s when Miller demonstrated a link between reduced hospital admissions for ketoacidosis and hypoglycaemia and diabetes education. A great deal of research has been undertaken since then, which suggests knowledge is important; however, knowledge alone is not enough to encourage people to engage in effective self-care. An effective therapeutic relationship is a key determining factor.

Many educators assume people newly diagnosed with diabetes know very little about diabetes and require rigorous detailed diabetes education to overcome their knowledge deficits to be able to undertake self-care. In fact, many people with diabetes have some information about the disease, have developed an explanatory model to explain *their* diabetes and sought 'facts' about the disease. These explanatory models and 'facts' may be very different from those of educators: in fact they usually are, but they are no less 'true'. Educators often regard people's explanatory models as myths to be dispelled rather than accepting them as part of the individual's story to be explored, discussed and understood.

Significantly, to the individual, diabetes is not 'failure of the pancreas to produce insulin', or 'insulin that does not work properly' that needs to be 'addressed', 'managed', 'treated', 'fixed' or 'cured'. It is an emotional as well as physical presence that affects the individual's whole being for the rest of their lives. Importantly, the physical aspects of people's reactions cannot be separated from their emotional, social, economic and environmental circumstances. Thus, accepting diabetes and coping with the hard work of self-care for a lifetime has a significant impact and is part of the individual's personal journey. Most people do not make the journey alone, so involving family and other relevant carers is essential.

Although research has identified many commonalities in the way people react to diabetes diagnosis and their self-care behaviours, educators must never assume the commonality fits the person in front of them. They must strive to understand the individual's unique story and the social and environmental factors that shape their story.

In fact, psychosocial and environmental factors, including culture, support, health and other beliefs, fears, locus of control, effective communication and therapeutic relationship, may have a greater effect on outcomes than knowledge. Thus, the educator's social and emotional intelligence is as, or more, important than their knowledge of diabetes, the disease.

Many valid tools are available to measure these parameters—most of them focus on the person with diabetes, and success is largely concerned with whether the individual with diabetes' knowledge improves, they stay out of hospital and whether their blood pressure, HbA_{1c} and lipids are 'normal'. Education and clinical care largely focuses on changing the person with diabetes. Equal focus *must* be placed on changing/enhancing, and measuring, the educator's capacity to communicate, engage, empathise and engender hope: that is to effectively combine art and science.

Many models describe ways to help people with diabetes and optimal diabetes services. In addition, models such as the Health Belief Model, the Transtheoretical Model of Change and the Chronic Disease Model are widely used as the conceptual framework for diabetes education, service planning and research. However, few, if any, of these models help educators develop the skills to move from 'good' to 'exceptional' educators.

Diabetes care has come a long way, since it was first described as *diabetes maigre* (bad prognosis) and *diabetes gros* (big diabetes). Science and technology continue to make major contributions to our understanding of diabetes and produce new management options. However, the prime focus of this book is on exploring effective teaching and learning and suggesting how educators can continue to learn and grow professionally and personally, rather than on the disease, 'diabetes'.

The book is not concerned with what diabetes is, or medical care, and the focus is not on what people with diabetes need to know, or what they should be taught. Such information is clearly documented in many care standards, clinical practice guidelines and other publications. The book aims to encourage educators to reflect on their philosophy of diabetes education and how they teach.

Hopefully, the book will encourage educators to read widely, including fiction as well as clinical publications and evidence-based literature. Reading fiction enhances people's social and emotional intelligence. Debating about and reflecting on a broad range of topics can help educators understand themselves as well as people with diabetes. Significantly, educators are not immune from illness, including diabetes, which can affect the quality of their lives and how they teach and provide care.

Carl Rogers stated:

Relationships can't flourish if they do not operate in a climate of listening and non-judgmental acceptance of the other person's point of view. Empathy is the hallmark of a genuine person.

Rogers (1902–1987)

Trisha Dunning AM

Acknowledgements

Many people were inspirational during planning and writing this book. Most of the inspiration and challenges came from the people with diabetes I have been privileged to know since I began my journey as a diabetes educator in 1984—they were and continue to be my true teachers and a source of inspiration.

I am also grateful to the many fiction/creative writers whose great books help me reflect on how I behave in my personal and professional lives. These include the members of Geelong Writers and Deakin Literacy Society who critique my stories and poetry and share their life experiences and insights through their writing.

Many national and international colleagues shaped my thoughts about diabetes education over the years through formal discussions, committee work, clinical care, casual conversations and their contributions to diabetes education research.

I am grateful to my wonderful research team at Deakin University/ Barwon Health, Sally, Sue and Nicole, who understood my need to constantly scribble ideas in notebooks and endlessly discuss them and who managed to smile as they helped me track down references and sort out the table of contents.

I am, as always, indebted to my publishers, Wiley-Blackwell, for their enthusiastic response to the book proposal and their continued advice and support throughout the publication process. I especially thank Alexandra Mc Gregor who championed the book from the outset, Magenta Styles and Sarah Claridge for their advice and support, SPi Global who typeset the manuscript and the book cover designer, Garth Stewart.

Michelle Robins and I thank Diabetes Australia-Victoria and the Victorian Aboriginal Community Controlled Health Organisation (VACCHO) for permission to reproduce the Feltman teaching tool shown in Figure 10.1.

My thanks also go to the people who reviewed the book proposal and found it worthy of publication. I do not know who you are, but thank you.

Thanks are also due to Michelle Robins, Adjunct Professor Margaret McGill, Dr Sheridan Waldron, Dr Bodil Rasmussen, Dr Martha Funnell, Dr Seyda Ozcan, Eva Kan, Anne Belton, Anne Marie Felton, Dr Linda

Siminerio and Dr Ming Yeong Tan for providing a wealth of information on the questionnaire about leadership that is discussed in Chapter 13 and to the peer educators who shared their stories in Chapter 9—Rhonda Lee, Helen Thomasic, Norma Ryan and Millie Glinsky.

The book would not exist without the fabulous work and enthusiasm of the authors.

I am deeply grateful to Sir Michael Hirst, President Elect of the International Diabetes Federation, for agreeing to write the foreword and for writing such a great foreword despite being so busy.

Finally, my thanks go to my husband, John, my Westies, MacBeth and Bonnie, for their love, support and understanding when meals and walks were delayed so I could write just a few more lines, and my alpacas and chooks whose social interactions are a constant source of learning.

Trisha Dunning AM

List of Tables, Figures and Boxes

Tables

Figures

Boxes

List of Abbreviations

AE	Adverse event
CAM	Complementary and alternative therapies
DCCT	Diabetes Control and Complications Trial
DE	Diabetes educator
DKA	Diabetic ketoacidosis
FFA	Free fatty acids
FPG	Fasting plasma glucose
GDM	Gestational diabetes
GLM	Glucose lowering medicines
HbA_{1c}	Glycosylated haemoglobin
HP	Health professional
HRM	High risk medicine
IGT	Impaired glucose tolerance
LADA	Latent autoimmune diabetes in adults
MI	Myocardial infarct
OGTT	Oral glucose tolerance test
T1DM	Type 1 diabetes
T2DM	Type 2 diabetes
UKPDS	United Kingdom Prospective Diabetes Study
UTI	Urinary tract infection

1 Brief Overview of Diabetes, the Disease

Trisha Dunning AM

Deakin University and Barwon Health, Geelong, Victoria, Australia

The main goals of diabetes treatment are to prevent acute and long term complications and to improve quality of life (QOL) and avoid premature diabetes associated death.

Successful diabetes management relies on successful patient engagement as well as medical treatment, and regular assessment of education needs is as important as medical care.

Barrett (2011)

Introduction

Chapter 1 contains a brief outline of diabetes pathophysiology and diabetes management. It is the only place you will find these issues discussed in this book. Having a firm knowledge about these issues is essential for health professionals (HPs) to provide competent diabetes care. However, the main focus of the book is on the person with diabetes, not the disease, and encouraging HPs to reflect on and constantly evaluate their practice. These factors are encompassed in Barrett's (2011) second statement; however, holistic, individualised care is missing from the statement and these are essential to achieve optimal outcomes.

Overview of diabetes

Diabetes mellitus (diabetes) occurs when the body's capacity to utilise glucose, fat and protein is disturbed due to insulin deficiency or insulin resistance. If enough insulin is not produced or insulin action is defective, fat and protein stores are mobilised and converted into glucose to supply energy.

Diabetes Education: Art, Science and Evidence, First Edition. Edited by Trisha Dunning AM.
© 2013 John Wiley & Sons, Ltd. Published 2013 by John Wiley & Sons, Ltd.

However, fat metabolism requires insulin; therefore, insulin deficiency results in disordered fat metabolism and the intermediate products, ketone bodies, accumulate in the blood and cause ketosis, especially in type 1 diabetes (T1DM). Mobilisation of protein stores leads to weight loss and weakness and causes lethargy.

Different types of diabetes have different underlying causal mechanisms and present differently. Generally, young people are insulin-deficient and have T1DM and older people are insulin-resistant and have type 2 diabetes (T2DM). However, the classification of diabetes is not made according to age. T1DM occurs in about 10% of older people often as latent autoimmune diabetes (LADA). Likewise, T2DM is becoming more prevalent in children and adolescents as a consequence of inactivity, obesity and genetic predisposition (Barr et al. 2005; Zimmet et al. 2007). In addition, beta cell failure occurs gradually in T2DM with consequent insulin deficiency; therefore, more than 50% of people with T2DM eventually require insulin (UKPDS 1998). T2DM is the most common type, over 85% of diagnosed people, and approximately 15% of diagnosed people have T1DM. However, there are cultural variations in the prevalence of the two types (EURODIAB ACE Study Group 2000; DIAMOND Project Group 2006; Soltesz et al. 2006).

Prevalence of diabetes

Diabetes affects approximately 0.5–10% of the population depending on the diabetes type, age and ethnic group. Diabetes prevalence is increasing, particularly in the older people and in developing countries. In Western countries, the overall prevalence is 4–6% and up to 10–12% among 60–70-year-olds. The prevalence rises to ~20% in developing countries (Diabetes Atlas 2011). Most countries spend 6–12% of their annual health budgets on diabetes and its consequences. Most of the morbidity and mortality is associated with T2DM.

Overview of normal glucose homeostasis

Glucose homeostasis refers to the delicate balance between the fed and the fasting states and is maintained by several interrelated hormones, especially insulin, glucagon, adrenalin, cortisol, and the incretins, and nutritional status including liver and muscle glucose stores, the type of food consumed, exercise type and regularity, and tissue sensitivity to insulin. Insulin action is mediated via two protein pathways: protein 13-kinase through the insulin receptors in cells, which influences glucose uptake into the cells, and MAP-kinase, which stimulates growth and mitogenesis.

Insulin is secreted in two phases: In the first-phase, insulin secretion begins within 2 min of nutrient ingestion and continues for 10–15 min. A second phase of insulin secretion follows the first phase and is sustained until normoglycaemia is restored. The first phase demonstrates insulin sensitivity and beta cell responsiveness to a glucose load. The first phase helps limit the post-prandial rise in blood glucose. It is diminished or lost in T2DM; consequently, post-prandial blood glucose levels are often elevated (Dornhorst 2001). Post-prandial hyperglycaemia plays a leading role in the development of atherosclerosis, hypertriglyceridaemia, coagulopathies, endothelial dysfunction and hypertension. Together with chronic hyperglycaemia, these factors are responsible for long-term diabetes complications (Ceriello 2000).

A number of factors contribute to hyperglycaemia:

- Impaired glucose utilisation (IGT)
- Reduced glucose storage
- Inadequately suppressed glucose-mediated hepatic glucose production
- High fasting glucose (FPG)
- Reduced post-prandial glucose utilisation

In turn, hyperglycaemia leads to elevated free fatty acids (FFAs), which inhibit insulin signalling and glucose transport, but FFAs are a source of metabolic fuel for the heart and liver.

Signs and symptoms of diabetes

T1DM usually presents with the so-called classic symptoms of diabetes mellitus:

- Polyuria
- Polydipsia
- Lethargy
- Weight loss
- Hyperglycaemia
- Glycosuria
- Blood and urinary ketones; sometimes the person presents in diabetic ketoacidosis (DKA), a serious life-threatening emergency. DKA also develops during illnesses in T1DM. Insulin is essential to prevent DKA and increased doses are often required during illness. In hospital settings, insulin is usually administered in an intravenous insulin infusion.

T2DM is an insidious progressive disease that is often diagnosed when the person presents with a diabetes complication such as neuropathy, cardiovascular disease, nephropathy or retinopathy, or when the individual consults a HP for an illness or during health screening programmes. It is not 'just a touch of sugar' or 'mild diabetes'. In fact, T2DM is also known as 'the silent killer', because the individual may not notice any symptoms. Therefore, population screening and education programmes are essential to enable early diagnosis and management.

The symptoms of T2DM are often less obvious than in T1DM; however, once T2DM diabetes is diagnosed and treatment is commenced, people often state they have more energy and feel less thirsty. Other signs of T2DM, especially in older people, include recurrent *Candida* infections, incontinence, constipation, dehydration and cognitive changes.

People most at risk of developing T2DM:

- Are overweight: abdominal obesity, increased body mass index (BMI), and a high waist–hip ratio. The specific parameters for these factors differ among some ethnic groups.
- Binge eating often precedes T2DM and contributes to obesity; however, the prevalence of eating disorders is similar in T1 and T2 diabetes (Herpertz et al. 1998).
- Are over age 40; but note there is increasing prevalence of T2DM in younger people.
- Have close relatives with T2DM.
- Are women who had gestational diabetes (GDM) or large babies.
- Currently smoke or smoked in the past (Kong et al. 2007).
- Are hypertensive, which is an independent predictor of T2DM (Conen et al. 2007).
- Insulin deficiency could be partly due to the enzyme PKC epsilon (PKCe), which is activated by fat, and inhibits insulin production (Biden 2007).

The majority of people with T2DM require multiple therapies to achieve and maintain acceptable blood glucose and lipid targets over the first 9 years after diagnosis (UKPDS 1998). Between 50% and 70% require insulin, which is often used in combination with oral glucose lowering medicines (GLM). This means diabetes management becomes progressively more complicated for people and increases the risk of medicine-related errors and adverse events as well as medicine non-compliance (see Chapter 11). The self-care regimen often becomes more demanding when the person is older, when their ability to self-manage may be compromised, which increases the likelihood of non-compliance and the costs of managing the disease for both the patient and the health system.

Gestational diabetes

Diabetes occurring during pregnancy is referred to as gestational diabetes (GDM). GDM causes varying degrees of carbohydrate intolerance that first occurs or is first recognised during pregnancy. GDM occurs in 1–14%

of pregnancies. The exact cause of GDM is unknown, but several factors are implicated including the same factors that predispose people to T2DM, as well as the number of previous pregnancies, previous large babies and short stature (Langer 2006).

Diagnosing diabetes

T1DM usually presents with symptoms, especially rapid weight loss, thirst and polyuria. A blood glucose test confirms the diagnosis. Sometimes C-peptide, a marker of insulin production, and islet cell antibodies (ICA), glutamic acid carboxylase (GAD) or tyrosine phosphatase (IA-2A) antibody tests are performed. Some or all of these antibodies are present in 85% of people with T1DM.

T2DM may also present with symptoms of hyperglycaemia and the diagnosis can be confirmed by laboratory blood glucose testing where a random plasma glucose >11.1 mmol/L and symptoms are diagnostic of T2DM. If the person is asymptomatic, fasting blood glucose >7 mmol/L on at least two occasions is required to confirm the diagnosis. Some guidelines indicate the diagnosis can be made if blood glucose is >6.5 mmol/L (American Diabetes Association (ADA)). The ADA does not advocate routine oral glucose tolerance test (OGTT) on the basis that the revised fasting level is sensitive enough to detect most people at risk of diabetes. Australia supports the continued use of the OGTT when the diagnosis is equivocal and to detect GDM (Hilton et al. 2002; Twigg et al. 2007).

Hyperglycaemia is a common stress response to serious intercurrent illness such as cardiovascular disease and infection, and it can be difficult to diagnose diabetes in such circumstances. However, it is important to control the blood glucose during illness to prevent adverse outcomes, including in non-diabetics. Although people with T2DM rarely develop DKA, they can develop hyperglycaemic, hyperosmolar states (HHS), which still have a high morbidity and mortality rate. Diabetes can present for the first time as HHS in undiagnosed older people.

Other screening and prevention measures include providing the public with information about diabetes, health maintenance programmes, and self-risk assessment tools, for example the Agency for Healthcare Research and Quality (AHRQ), risk tools which are available on the Internet (from http://www.ahrq.gov/ppip/helthywom.htm or http://www.ahrq.gov/ppip/helthymen.htm) and The Australian Type 2 Diabetes Risk Assessment Tool (AUSDRISK) (Diabetes Australia 2010).

The place of HbA_{1c} as a diagnostic tool is still debated. High HbA_{1c} is a strong predictor of diabetes but not of cardiovascular disease after multivariate analysis and after excluding people diagnosed with diabetes within 2–5 years of follow-up (Pradhan et al. 2007). However, Pradhan et al. did not recommend using HbA_{1c} as a single predictor of diabetes risk. HbA_{1c} is a standard test for monitoring metabolic control.

Managing diabetes

Diabetes education and effective self-management are fundamental to achieving optimal diabetes management and outcomes. The value of diabetes education is described in numerous publications. However, diabetes is a complex, multifactorial disease and most people with diabetes, especially those with T2DM, require multiple therapies to manage the underlying pathophysiological changes and their consequences.

Likewise, diabetes treatment often becomes more complicated with increasing duration of diabetes. Thus, a collaborative interdisciplinary health-care team usually delivers diabetes care, and is considered best practice. However, the person with diabetes must play a key role in deciding their management and in undertaking self-care, see Chapter 10. HPs must provide relevant, timely individualised education to help the person, and often the person's carers undertake the demanding, lifelong, relentless role: diabetes self-care (see Chapters 2, 3, 5 and 6).

The person with diabetes is the most important member of the team followed by their family. Good communication among and between team members and with the person with diabetes/carers is essential to help ensure the individual that their family receives consistent information. Communication might include guidelines and well-defined care pathways. Likewise, it is imperative that information about the individual is shared between and within hospital departments and other health services to facilitate smooth transitions among services.

The diabetes team usually consists of some or all of the following:

- Diabetologist
- Diabetes nurse specialist/diabetes educator and/or diabetes nurse practitioner
- Dietitian
- Podiatrist
- Social worker
- Psychologist
- General practitioner

Other professionals who contribute regularly to diabetes care include the following:

- Ophthalmologist
- Optometrist
- Vascular specialists, orthopaedic surgeons, neurologists, urologists and dentists
- Cultural health workers, for example Australian Aboriginal health workers and traditional healers in Africa
- Exercise physiologists
- Physiotherapists

In addition, hospital staff who care for people in hospital become team members during hospital and emergency room admissions, including the following:

- Doctors
- Nurses
- Dietitians
- Physiotherapists
- Occupational therapists
- Audiologists (Dunning 2011)

Encouraging people to be actively engaged in their care, which includes determining the care goals and management regimen, is an essential responsibility of all team members. The relationship between the individual and HP is a significant determinant of care. While all team members must be skilled communicators, it is unrealistic to expect an individual to have close relationships with all team members.

HPs might regard the one who provides most of the advice and acts as the link among team members as the 'team leader'. However, most people with diabetes do not have the same concept of 'diabetes team care' as HPs. The HP the individual has the strongest relationship with might be the most effective team leader. The team needs to be supported by adequate resources, space and staff to perform optimally.

Diabetes management and management aims

Management aims are defined in a number of guidelines such as in the Australian Diabetes Society Position Statements, Clinical Management Guidelines for Diabetes in General Practice, and a range of self-management guidelines produced by various countries, for example The International Diabetes Federation Position Statements for T2DM, The UK *Diabetes National Service Framework: Standards* (2001), Diabetes Australia *Plan for a Better Life for People with Diabetes* (2004).

The basic aim defined in these guidelines is to maintain quality of life, keep the person free from diabetes symptoms, and prevent complications by controlling blood glucose, blood lipids and blood pressure with as few hypoglycaemic episodes as possible. Blood glucose range should be determined on an individual basis, usually between 3 and 6.5 mmol/L for 90% of tests, especially during acute illness and surgery, T1DM and young people with T2DM and during pregnancy. Regular complication screening and general health checks are very important. The latter include dental checks, mammograms, prostate checks and preventative vaccination, e.g. fluvax and pneumovax.

The regimen should affect the person's lifestyle and emotional well-being as little as possible, although some modification is usually necessary.

People with T1DM require regular insulin injections to survive. People with T2DM who are obese can sometimes be treated using a combination of diet and exercise, but people managed with diet are not monitored as carefully as those on medicines and have more hyperglycaemia and hypertension medicines (Hippisley-Cox and Pringle 2004).

As indicated, most people with T2DM require oral glucose lowering medicines and often eventually insulin. Individual needs must be considered and can only be known by undertaking a thorough history and physical examination and listening carefully to the individual's story. To achieve the latter, HPs must be expert listeners and be truly present in the consultation.

Empowerment care models and accepting people with diabetes' choices may mean the individual decides not to follow the HP's advice. Such a decision may or may not be in the individuals 'best interest' according the HP's risk criteria, but must be respected and not judged: the HP is responsible for ensuring the individual has all the information they require to make an informed decision. Information must be in a language and format they understand. The HP should check for understanding and document the episode carefully. These are the individual's rights. The decision about what to do with the information is the individual's prerogative and responsibility.

Long-term diabetes complications

The DCCT in 1993 and the UKPDS in 1998 demonstrated the relationship between the development and progression of diabetes' long-term complications in T1 and T2DM, respectively. The UKPDS also highlighted the fact that it is important to control blood pressure to reduce the risk of cardiovascular disease. The main long-term complications are as follows:

- Macrovascular disease:
  - Myocardial infarction
  - Cerebrovascular accident
  - Intermittent claudication
- Microvascular disease associated with thickening of the basement membranes of the small blood vessels, e.g.:
  - Retinopathy
  - Nephropathy, which leads to anaemia and its consequences including tiredness
- Neuropathy or damage to the autonomic and peripheral nerves:
  - Peripheral: reduced sensation in hands and especially the feet, which can lead to ulcers, Charcot's arthropathy and amputation
  - Autonomic: erectile dysfunction, atonic bladder and urine retention, and gastroparesis

- Complications of pregnancy, which can affect the mother and/or the baby:
  - Mother: toxaemia, polyhydramnous intrauterine death, Caesarean section
  - Baby: congenital abnormalities, premature birth, respiratory distress, hypoglycaemia at birth
- Emotional distress, depression and burnout

Other complications also occur in the long term and need to be monitored. These include hearing loss, dental disease, some forms of cancer associated with obesity, and concomitant endocrine disease. For example, T1DM is an autoimmune disease and people with T1DM have a greater risk of developing other autoimmune diseases such as coeliac disease and hyperthyroidism.

A number of other factors appear to contribute to the development of diabetic complications. These include free radicals (ROS), advanced glycated end products (AGE), changes in cellular signalling and endothelial humoral components that affect coagulation and increase the likelihood of microthrombi.

All HPs who care for a person with diabetes are responsible for monitoring complications status and the effects of complications on their self-care potential and negotiating with the individual to revise the management plan. A full complication assessment should be undertaken at least every 12 months. HPs need to proactively identify opportunities for health and complication screening and education, that is recognise 'the teachable moment'.

Summary

Diabetes is a complex, changeable and challenging condition. Medical management is essential but must be combined with effective education that enhances the individual's and their family's self-care capacity. The latter depends on effective communication and respect.

References

American Diabetes Association, American Psychiatric Association, American Association of Clinical Endocrinologists, North American Association for the Study of Obesity. (2004) Consensus development conference on antipsychotic drugs and obesity and diabetes. *Diabetes Care* 27: 596–601.

Barr EL, Magliano DJ, Zimmet PZ et al. (2005) *The Australian Diabetes, Obesity and Lifestyle Study (AusDiab). Tracking the Accelerating Epidemic: Its Causes and Outcomes.* Melbourne, Victoria, Australia, International Diabetes Institute.

Barrett A. (2011) Ensuring high quality structured education for people with diabetes. *Diabetes and Primary Care* 13(3): 178.

Biden T. (2007) Major breakthrough in understanding type 2 diabetes. Interview in *Nursing Review* November 2007: 10.

Ceriello A. (2000) The postprandial state and cardiovascular disease: relevance to diabetes mellitus. *Diabetes Metabolism Research Reviews* 16: 125–132.

Conen D, Ridker P, Mora S et al. (2007) Blood pressure and risk of developing type 2 diabetes mellitus: The Women's Health Study. *European Heart Journal* 28(23): 2937–2943.

Diabetes and Control and Complications Trial Research Group. (1993) The effect of intensive insulin treatment on the development and progression of long term complications of insulin dependent diabetes. *New England Journal of Medicine* 329: 977–986.

Diabetes Australia. (2010) *Australian Type 2 Diabetes Risk Assessment Tool (AUSDRISK)*. http://www.diabetesaustralia.org.au (accessed July 2011).

DIAMOND Project Group. (2006) Incidence and trends of childhood type 1 diabetes worldwide 1990–1999. *Diabetic Medicine* 23: 857–866.

Dornhorst A. (2001) Insulinotrophic meglitinide analogues. *Lancet* 358(9294): 1709–1716.

Dunning T. (2011) What is 'the diabetes health-care team?' *Diabetes Conquest* Autumn: 12–13.

EURODIAB ACE Study Group. (2000) Variation and trends in incidence of childhood diabetes in Europe. *Lancet* 355: 873–876.

EURODIAB Substudy 2 Study Group. (2000) Vitamin D supplement in early childhood and risk for Type 1 (insulin-dependent) diabetes mellitus. *Diabetologia* 42(1): 51–54.

Herpertz S, Albus C, Wagener R. (1998) Cormorbidity of eating disorders. Does diabetes control reflect disturbed eating behaviour? *Diabetes Care* 21(7): 1110–1116.

Hilton D, O'Rourke P, Welbourn T, Reid, C. (2002) Diabetes detection in Australian general practice: a comparison of diagnostic criteria. *Medical Journal of Australia* 176: 104–107.

Hippisley-Cox J, Pringle M. (2004) Diabetics treated with diet only have more complications. *Lancet*. http://www.medscape.com/viewarticle/484479 5.8.2004

International Diabetes Federation (IDF). (2006) The IDF consensus worldwide definition of the metabolic syndrome. IDF, Brussels (accessed December 2007).

International Diabetes Federation (IDF). (2011) *IDF Diabetes Atlas*, 5th edn. Brussels, Belgium, International Diabetes Federation.

Kong A, Williams R, Smith M et al. (2007) *Acanthosis nigricans* and diabetes risk factors: prevalence in young persons seen in southwestern US primary care practices. *Annals of Family Medicine* 5(3): 202–208.

Langer O. (2006) Management of gestational diabetes: pharmacological treatment options and glycaemic control. *Endocrinology Metabolism Clinics of North America* 35: 53–78.

Pradhan A, Rifai N, Buring J, Ridker P. (2007) Hemoglobin A1c predicts diabetes but not cardiovascular disease in nondiabetic women. *The American Journal of Medicine* 120(8): 720–727.

Soltesz G, Patterson C, Dahlquist G. (2006) Global trends in childhood obesity, in: *Diabetes Atlas*, 3rd edn. Brussels, Belgium, International Diabetes Federation (IDF), pp. 154–190.

Twigg S, Kamp M, Davis T et al. (2007) Prediabetes: a position statement from the Australian Diabetes Society and Australian Diabetes Educators Association. *Medical Journal of Australia* 186(9): 461–465.

UKPDS (United Kingdom Prospective Diabetes Study). (1998) Intensive blood glucose control with sulphonylureas or insulin compared with conventional treatment and risk of complications in patients with type 2 diabetes (UKPDS 33). *Lancet* 352: 837–853.

Zimmet P, Alberti G, Kaufman F, et al. (2007) The metabolic syndrome in children and adolescents – an IDF consensus report. *Paediatric Diabetes* 8: 299–306.

2 The Journey of the Person with Diabetes

Jane Speight[1,2,3] and Harsimran Singh[4]

[1] *The Australian Centre for Behavioural Research in Diabetes, Diabetes Australia, Melbourne, Victoria, Australia*
[2] *Centre for Mental Health and Well-being Research, School of Psychology, Deakin University, Geelong, Victoria, Australia*
[3] *AHP Research, Hornchurch, Essex, UK*
[4] *Department of Neurobehavioural Sciences, Behavioural Medicine Centre, School of Medicine, University of Virginia, Charlottesville, Virginia, USA*

> *The road of life twists and turns and no two directions are ever the same.*
> *Yet our lessons come from the journey, not the destination.*
>
> Don Williams Jr. (1957–)

Introduction

The experience of living with diabetes is, inevitably, different for everyone who lives with the condition: a unique journey shaped by many factors, including type of diabetes, age at diagnosis, treatment regimen, prior health status, personality, emotional reaction, and social circumstance. The analogy of living with diabetes as a journey helps health professionals understand the distinctive quality of that experience. There will be times when the person feels well and copes positively and other times that are more challenging, when resilience can be tested. There is no single successful route health professionals can recommend for all people with diabetes—there will be detours, delays, potholes and speed bumps along the way based on the personal and clinical circumstances of each person.

Along the journey, the person can be assisted and supported by others who help read the map. Alternatively, the individual can be harassed by 'backseat drivers' who offer conflicting, erroneous or unwanted suggestions. Thus, family, friends, and health professionals can be a source of support or conflict. In this chapter, we do not attempt to map out the 'typical' journey: instead, we provide insights into how the journey might be

---

experienced by some people with diabetes and, importantly, point out signposts that could help you to recognise when support is needed and how to provide it.

From a biomedical perspective, diabetes is a chronic disease—it has a pathology, various aspects of which can be investigated in the laboratory. However, in this chapter (indeed in the book) you will not read much about diabetes the disease. Instead, we are interested in the human experience of diabetes: how individuals perceive diabetes, cope with it, live with it and what health professionals can learn from each individual's experience to support other people living with diabetes.

Although understanding the pathology is necessary, it is not sufficient to ensure successful clinical and patient-reported outcomes. Understandably, health professionals are likely to guide diabetes management from a biomedical perspective, yet the persons' self-care decisions and behaviours are likely to be influenced by their own experiences, beliefs, responsibilities, and preferences (Adams et al. 1997). Thus, understanding people's experience of living with diabetes is fundamental to effectively supporting people along their journey (Telford et al. 2006).

Numerous studies present snapshots of the impact of diabetes on people's physical and psychological circumstances at certain life stages or life transitions. However, there is a dearth of research about how people experience their journey with diabetes, for example from diagnosis to when they feel in control of their diabetes or, in other cases, entirely overpowered by it. A few qualitative studies have highlighted the complex personal experiences and insights that a person gains on their journey with diabetes. In a study of 13 people with a recent diagnosis of diabetes, Kneck et al. (2011) identified four common themes:

- Being 'taken over by a new reality', e.g. concrete changes are necessary as a result of diabetes.
- 'The body plays a new role in life', e.g. the body has new demands and the blood glucose metre becomes a valuable tool to better understand these requirements.
- 'Different ways of learning', e.g. experience and reflection become useful learning tools.
- 'The healthcare services as a necessary partner', e.g. health professionals are perceived as a source of reliable information.

Even this brief summary highlights the reality of the issues people face as they begin their journey with diabetes. People gain an understanding of diabetes through their own experiences and self-reflection, and they grapple with a new reality that involves changing perceptions of their own body, lifestyle and the future. Thus, it is evident that psychological, social and behavioural factors play a vital role in the person's journey with diabetes.

Psychological factors: the role of beliefs and attitudes

When an individual develops an acute condition, there is usually a sudden onset of symptoms, a short period of treatment and, hopefully, a relatively speedy recovery. While definitions of 'chronicity' vary in terms of the extent of disability, pain and intensity of the care required, the common human experience of diabetes is that its course is unclear and unrelenting. The onset can be different depending on the type of diabetes. It can be sudden, as is most frequently the case in type 1 diabetes (T1DM) and gestational diabetes (GDM) or silent and insidious as is often the case with type 2 diabetes (T2DM). Diabetes can be detected when symptoms develop, the severity and type of the symptoms, when a complication develops, or come 'out of the blue' on routine screening. The following quotations from people with diabetes illustrate how the impact of the diagnosis can be influenced by personal experience and how attitudes begin to take shape:

- *'When I was first diagnosed it was very dramatic, it was really frightening, the fear of the unknown really.'*
- *'I don't think it's all that devastating. There are far worse incurable sorts of things.'*
- *'It was easy for me because my son had it, so I had the experience of it, I knew what it was already.'*

Clark (2004, p. 29)

At the beginning of any journey, especially if it is long and complicated, we need a map or at least some decent directions to put us on the right road. At the beginning of their journeys, people with diabetes need clear directions from their health professionals about the diagnosis, as well as an explanation of the condition and its management. Giving the right information, the right amount of information, at the right time, and in the right way is crucial to ensure the individual 'begins the journey on the right track'.

Qualitative studies indicate health professionals need to inform people with diabetes that diabetes care is a process and clearly explain what the care process will look like so the person has a 'map' to help them on their journey. Indeed, the way diabetes is diagnosed and the information given at that critical teachable moment influences the way people perceive their condition for many years to come. Clarity, timing and the authority with which the diagnosis is made are highly salient for people with newly diagnosed type 2 diabetes (Parry et al. 2004).

Delays confirming the diagnosis, referring the individual to specialists, and creating management plans all contribute to the individual being unclear about the diagnosis and the need for lifestyle changes. Some people felt they were 'in limbo' waiting for the formal diagnosis after the initial clinical tests, particularly people with no symptoms or obvious signs of diabetes. Many people interpret the lack of symptoms as evidence they do not have diabetes or that it is so 'mild' it does not warrant urgent attention. Furthermore, a large UK quantitative study demonstrated that 46% of people with newly diagnosed T2DM did not believe diabetes was 'a serious threat to their health' (Khunti et al. 2008).

In addition, people who indicated they understood their condition were more likely to report that it was long term and they could influence its course (Khunti et al. 2008). Thus, the period around the time diabetes is diagnosed represents an excellent opportunity for health professionals to intervene and equip the individual with adequate and clear information about what they need to know and do to make a confident start on their journey and learn to adapt appropriately to having diabetes.

Health beliefs are the foundations of motivation and differentiate between people who do and do not perform healthy behaviours (Cerkoney and Hart 1980; Gillibrand and Stevenson 2006). Systematic reviews indicate that 'adherence' to oral medications ranges from 36% to 93% in people with T2DM (Cramer 2004; DART Memo). Mann et al. (2009) investigated medication-taking behaviours, beliefs about diabetes and beliefs about medicines among 151 US adults with T2DM. One in four participants did not take their medications as recommended.

The following beliefs predicted the likelihood people would not take medicines as recommended:

- *'Believing you have diabetes only when your sugar is high'*
- *'believing there was no need to take medicine when the glucose was normal,'* *'worrying about side-effects of diabetes medicines'*
- *'lack of self-confidence to control diabetes'*
- *'feeling medicines are hard to take'.*

Mann et al. (2009)

A meta-analysis indicated that people who are more likely to take their medications as recommended have a higher level of confidence in their ability to follow their health professionals' advice, expect more meaningful and positive consequences of their medication-taking behaviour, and view the relationship with their health professionals more positively (Gherman et al. 2011).

Furthermore, two other literature reviews demonstrated the way people think about their diabetes influences their outcomes. Hagger and Orbell's (2003) review of illness perceptions about diabetes and other chronic conditions found stronger beliefs that a condition is controllable were associated with greater psychological well-being, vitality and social functioning and were negatively associated with psychological distress and objective measures of illness status.

More recently, McSharry et ai. (2011) conducted a meta-analysis and systematic review regarding glycaemic control (HbA_{1c}) and illness perceptions in T1 and T2DM. They demonstrated that various illness perceptions were significantly related to HbA_{1c}. For example,

- Identity (i.e. symptoms attributed to diabetes),
- Consequences (i.e. beliefs about the effects of having diabetes),
- Timeline cyclical (i.e. course and duration of diabetes), and
- Emotional representation domains (i.e. affective responses to diabetes).

were all significantly and positively related to HbA_{1c}; in addition, a negative association between greater personal control and HbA_{1c} emerged. Thus, evidence is cumulating that indicates personal beliefs about diabetes influence both psychological and biomedical outcomes.

'Psychological insulin resistance' (PIR) is characterised by a general reluctance among people with T2DM to initiate insulin therapy (Polonsky 2004; Brod et al. 2009) and can pose a significant threat to overall diabetes management. Polonsky (2004), who first coined the term 'psychological insulin resistance', suggested PIR is caused by several factors:

- Perceived loss of control—61% believe 'once I start insulin, I can never stop', 50% believe insulin will restrict their lives.
- Poor self-efficacy—up to 50% did not believe they could handle the demands of insulin.
- Perceived personal failure—up to 50% believe 'if I have to take insulin, it means that I have messed up, that I haven't done a good enough job taking care of my diabetes'.
- Perceived disease severity—many people believe requiring insulin means their diabetes is suddenly much more serious or has got worse or, indeed, that it will get worse because of insulin. Polonsky cited a large ethnic split on this issue; around 70% of Hispanics believed diabetes became more serious versus 8% of non-Hispanics.
- Injection-related anxiety—approximately 50% are scared of injections, although the proportion seems to be overstated. Very few people actually have needle phobia. Being scared is more likely to be due to lack of awareness about the relative painlessness of insulin injections.
- Perceived lack of positive gain—less than 10% believe insulin will have benefits for energy and blood glucose levels.

You may notice only one of these factors; injection-related anxiety is an emotional reaction and even that is likely to have its basis in mistaken beliefs. The other factors are all beliefs and attitudes. In other words, the way people think about diabetes affects how they are willing to manage it. Consider the following personal account (Box 2.1):

My mother had diabetes, and it was no big deal to her for over 20 years. She rarely saw a doctor and never paid much attention to it, and it never really

---

> **Box 2.1   Personal accounts of the diagnosis of diabetes**
>
> Member of the teen-sensation musical band 'Jonas Brothers', Nick Jonas, has discussed the time around the diagnosis of his type 1 diabetes in 2005 when he was 12 years old (von Wartburg 2007). A few weeks before his diagnosis, he noticed he was losing a considerable amount of weight, was continually thirsty and generally having a bad attitude—'it was just insane. I had a terrible attitude, which was totally odd for me because I'm actually a nice person. Especially being on the road around people all the time, you have to keep that positive energy going … and it was hard.' His blood sugar was over 700 mg/DL (39 mmol/L) on diagnosis and he said, 'to suddenly have the shock of diabetes was a bit overwhelming in itself, and then I had to learn all about it, learn all these things in such a short period of time. All of it was crazy. I also wondered if I could continue making music….'
>
> Professional V8 Supercar racing driver, Jack Perkins, described his experience of being diagnosed with type 1 diabetes (www.sweet-talkdiabetes.com). He said he was 'living the dream' as a professional racing driver when he was diagnosed with type 1 diabetes in 2006 and was told he 'would never race again'. He said 'I was shattered at first, thinking all my plans for the future were destroyed'.

bothered her. But then her doctor finally convinced her to start insulin and— bam! Over the next year, she started having serious problems with her eyes, and then there were terrible pains in her legs. In fact, she eventually lost most of her left leg. No doubt about it, insulin was the culprit. And now you want me to start insulin? No way!

Polonsky (2004, p. 148)

Finally, Polonsky indicated health professionals' attitudes and language are important in shaping the individual's willingness to initiate insulin. All too often, health professionals use insulin as a threat by talking with the individual about their need to 'improve your lifestyle or start insulin'. Many health professionals also refer to 'failure' of lifestyle changes or oral medications. While these phrases may seem harmless and even motivational messages, the individual interprets the underlying meaning as: 'you have failed; your diabetes has got worse, now you have to pay the price'. Refer to Chapter 6 for more information about the importance of language when communicating with and about people with diabetes and Chapter 11 for more information about medicine-related beliefs and behaviours.

These studies highlight the various 'teaching moments' around the time of diagnosis that can be used constructively to help people with diabetes understand their condition better and the journey they are embarked on.

Diabetes educators and other health professionals can use simple cognitive restructuring techniques to develop appropriate health beliefs among people with diabetes. For example, blood glucose 'tests', regardless of whether they are conducted at home or as part of routine clinic visits, e.g. HbA_{1c}, can lead to anxiety and feelings of self-blame especially if the individual learned to interpret high blood glucose as 'failing a test' or a 'poor reading' (Peel et al. 2004) and can lead to less frequent blood glucose self-monitoring (SMBG) and missed clinic appointments (Karter et al. 2004; Weinger et al. 2005).

Health professionals can help people with diabetes use SMBG as an opportunity to help them understand how their blood glucose levels respond to their medication, diet, physical activity, and how to use their SMBG readings to maintain or make changes to their self-care regimen and feel more empowered to influence the course of their condition (Peel et al. 2007). Aiming for consistently perfect blood glucose readings is unrealistic. The reading is not a 'test' of the individual's performance: it is an opportunity to help the individual decide what to do next, e.g. 'is it safe to drive?', 'how much insulin do I need?', 'do I need a snack to avoid a hypo?'

Beliefs about diabetes and its severity often arise from information about diabetes-related complications. Indeed, many health professionals use the threat of complications as a motivational tool, intentionally or otherwise. 'Worrying about the future and the possibility of serious complications' ranks as the number one concern of people with diabetes, regardless of diabetes type, and is consistent across cultures (Snoek et al. 2000). The threat of long-term complications emerged as a strong motivator to encourage children to engage in better self-care in a qualitative study involving 47 caregivers of children with type 1 diabetes (parents and others) that focused on acquiring information from health professional. One parent commented that it was the only tool they had to motivate children: 'the hammer we have, and the only hammer, is long-term complications' (Buckloh et al. 2008).

However, people with diabetes typically overestimate their risk of complications (Asimakopoulou et al. 2008), which can have a counter-intuitive effect on motivation to prevent or delay the onset of complication. People become side-tracked into managing their emotional reactions such as anxiety and depression rather than actively managing their risk factors. Furthermore, people with diabetes tend to underestimate the value of lifestyle changes and taking medications as recommended to prevent the onset of complications. They typically rate 'getting regular medical tests' to screen for complications as a more important preventative strategy than self-care behaviours (Skinner 2004). Thus, is it clear that beliefs and attitudes formed before diabetes was diagnosed and those formed around the time of diagnosis, or later in the journey with diabetes, influence the way people manage their diabetes and, to a large extent, the path their diabetes will take.

Psychological factors: emotional reactions to diabetes

Diabetes has physical and psychological consequences. Most people battle with diabetes at some point in their lives: some are angry, others depressed, some are guilt-ridden, others in denial, some are frustrated, others frightened. Diabetes is not simply a matter of eating the 'right' things, avoiding the 'wrong' things and taking medications as recommended. It is an emotional journey. Indeed, overcoming emotional reactions is likely to be one of the most important steps a person can take to manage their diabetes success-fully. Yet, it is singularly the most overlooked aspect of diabetes care. Time and money is spent on screening for retinopathy and other complications of diabetes, and yet, very little effort is put into screening for emotional distress.

Significantly the severity of depressed mood is associated with less healthy diet and fewer medication-taking behaviours as well as functional impairment and higher healthcare costs (Ciechanowski et al. 2000). Estimates vary, but systematic reviews suggest as many as 20% of the people with diabetes could have clinically significant levels of depression—up to four times higher than the general population (Ali et al. 2006; Barnard et al. 2006). Many more people, an estimated 40%, experience poor psychological well-being (Peyrot et al. 2005) including diabetes-related distress. Diabetes-related distress refers to emotional distress caused by or about the experience of diabetes and its management.

These facts mean that one in every five people with diabetes you see is likely to be depressed, and almost every other person could be experiencing severe diabetes-related distress. Can you identify these people in your clinic? Perhaps not; but you are not alone. Health professionals only identify and document one in four people with severe distress in routine consultations (Pouwer et al. 2006), which suggests detecting emotional distress is problematic unless routine, systematic monitoring is imple-mented using brief, standardised, valid measures.

Similarly, a cross-national study found 25% of people with diabetes reported symptoms indicating likely depression or diabetes-related dis-tress (5% had both) and 80% of these were newly identified (Snoek et al. 2011). In the only study in which people experiencing high levels of psychological distress related to their diabetes were asked whether they wanted to talk with a health professional about their concerns, high concordance was noted between needing and wanting to talk (Davies et al. 2006).

So, along the journey with diabetes, it is almost certain that the indi-vidual will hit some hurdles—the reality of the diagnosis, changes in the treatment regimen, the onset of complications, as well as general life tran-sitions and stresses such as becoming pregnant, moving house. All of these transitions can, and usually do, evoke emotional responses. Be aware that emotions are an inherent part of human experience and a natural response to the stresses of managing diabetes every day.

Recognising emotional problems can be difficult because people with diabetes do not always recognise their own complex feelings or may be too embarrassed to discuss their emotions with a health professional. Simple questioning techniques can be used to ensure the individual realises they are not abnormal because they feel the way they do. Some useful questions include:

- 'Everyone struggles with their diabetes from time-to-time. What is that like for you?'
- 'How can I help you get past some of the difficulties you are experiencing?'

See Box 2.2 for other question suggestions.

Health professionals face three main challenges when they address emotional issues during consultations: discomfort, feeling the need to solve the 'problems', and time. Often, health professionals avoid opening the emotional 'can of worms' because they fear they do not have the skills to deal with an emotional outburst (Mosely et al. 2010). Discussing emotional difficulties and 'problem areas' should be regarded as an opportunity for health professionals to learn about the individual's journey.

Health professionals do not need to solve the problems or change the person's emotions. Their role is to create an environment in which emotional reactions are valid and can be expressed freely. Frequently, the person just wants an opportunity to express their frustrations, guilt, or anger and have their feelings validated by their health professional. Furthermore, the time taken to listen to individual's frustrations is well spent because it illuminates the human experience and can provide insights into why the person manages their diabetes the way they do.

Box 2.2   A few example questions that can be used to explore how the person is faring on their journey with diabetes

- What is the hardest thing for you right now about living with diabetes?
- What would you like us to talk about today?
- You obviously work hard at managing your diabetes, what is your reason for working so hard?
- Diabetes can drive people crazy. What really gets to you about having diabetes?
- What worries you most about living with diabetes?
- How do you feel about the way your family members participate in your diabetes management? What would you like to change?
- What self-care skills would you like to improve?
- How would you like things to turn out for you in 2 years?

Social factors: influence of personal situation

Diabetes has been referred to as a 'family disease' (Anderson et al. 1981) because the clinical and patient-reported outcomes of people with diabetes, including their overall adjustment to the condition, is largely related to how they manage their diabetes in daily life outside the clinic environment (Fisher et al. 1998). This is especially true for children and adolescents with diabetes because most of their diabetes care is provided by their parents and families. However, this can be equally true of older men from certain ethnic groups; for example, meals are prepared by a wife or daughter in some cultures (Singh et al. submitted).

Various treatment models such as the 'Family Approach to Diabetes Management', which involves significant others from a child's family and focuses on emotional supportiveness within the family, family organisation/communication patterns, and competence, have been applied successfully with this population leading to favourable clinical and patient-reported outcomes (Hanson et al. 1995; Anderson et al. 1999; Solowiejczyk 2004).

Studies involving adults with diabetes consistently show the need to recognise the family context in which the condition is managed and integrate significant others when developing a management plan with the individual (Delamater et al. 2001; Chesla et al. 2003). Strong family networks are an essential feature of various ethnic communities and are an important source of information as well as emotional support for the person with diabetes, e.g. among South Asians (Brar 2005; Stone et al. 2005) and African-Americans (Samuel-Hodge et al. 2000). Likewise, higher levels of perceived family support and greater self-efficacy are associated with higher reported levels of diet and exercise self-care by Mexican-Americans with diabetes (Wen et al. 2004).

However, it is important to note that 'family' may not always act as a support system and may, in fact, sometimes be a barrier to optimal diabetes care (Maillet et al. 1996). Families may impose their socio-cultural beliefs regarding illness, thereby making it difficult for the individual to perform the recommended self-care behaviours. In other words, if healthcare recommendations are not consistent with the beliefs and value of the individual's significant others, it is likely to impact their self-management of the condition and can cause family conflict.

Given the complex relationships that exist between people with diabetes and their families, friends and colleagues, it is important for health professionals to understand the role of the individual's family context in their diabetes management. It may be appropriate to encourage family members to attend some clinic appointments. Their attendance could help ensure both the person with diabetes and their family have a shared understanding of the most suitable ways to manage the condition.

Social stigma surrounding diabetes is prevalent in certain ethnic groups and appears to be growing in society as a whole (Schabert et al. submitted). For example, there is significant cultural pressure on younger South Asian men and women with diabetes to hide their condition from others (Ramachandran et al. 2005; Singh et al. submitted). Unsurprisingly, such pressure can make diabetes self-management harder and more complex, which in extreme cases can lead to the individual concealing their condition in public. At the least, it can result in instances of delayed or missed insulin injections, SMBG or taking medication.

In more extreme cases, cultural pressure can have dire long-term consequences. Goenka et al. (2004) presented a case report of a British South Asian girl with T2DM. Both the girl and her family refused to accept any treatment for her diabetes despite the fact that her mother had insulin-treated T2DM, because they felt accepting the diagnosis of diabetes would hinder her marriage prospects. The girl developed severe microvascular complications before she finally agreed to treat her diabetes. Similar socio-cultural pressures surrounding illness have been observed in other cultures such as Vietnamese (Pham 2004).

Health disparities are evident in certain socioeconomic, cultural and older age groups due to the disproportionate burden of diabetes in these groups, which is compounded by lower levels of health literacy in these groups. Health literacy refers to an individual's ability to obtain, process, and understand health information and services needed to make appropriate health decisions (Selden et al. 2000). Among adults with T2DM, inadequate health literacy is associated with suboptimal HbA$_{1c}$ higher rates of retinopathy, even after adjusting for socio-demographic characteristics, depressive symptoms, social support, treatment regimen and duration of diabetes (Schillinger et al. 2002).

Thus, health literacy appears to contribute to the disproportionate burden of diabetes-related problems among people from certain social and cultural groups. It is essential, therefore, that health professionals ensure they communicate effectively (see Chapters 6 and 10) with people with diabetes and consider the various socio-demographic characteristics that could suggest suboptimal health literacy. It is, therefore, crucial to ensure messages are clearly explained but, most importantly, to check the person understands the message.

Factors that affect illness/wellness behaviours

Although it is impossible to predict how a person's journey with diabetes will unfold and at what points along the journey they might need more help and support, it is possible to highlight stages and transitions that many people with diabetes find challenging. We have attempted to highlight a few such signposts along the journey with diabetes when individuals could benefit from extra support from their diabetes care team, such as:

- The time of diagnosis
- Changing medication regimens e.g. oral to insulin; injections to pump
- When wanting family members to be more (or less) involved in diabetes care
- The onset of complications.

In addition, lifestyle changes such as modifying dietary patterns and physical activity are essential components of diabetes care that many people find extremely demanding and difficult to achieve (Wing et al. 2001). People with diabetes may resist lifestyle changes for various reasons such as not understanding how to make the change, why it is required, or because they do not have adequate support to make that change (Delamater, 2006).

Diabetes educators and other members of the clinical team can look out for resistance patterns in people with diabetes and encourage open dialogue with them to determine how to address the barriers to change. It is important to normalise people's experiences by acknowledging how difficult it can be to make such changes and to invite the person to indicate how they think they can best take small steps towards their goals. Motivational interviewing techniques have been used successfully to elicit 'change talk' (facilitating behaviour change) in people with diabetes who seem resistant to making the changes needed to optimise their diabetes care and, ultimately, their health outcomes (Welch et al. 2006).

Summary

In summary, it is clear that people experience diabetes in unique ways and that there is no single path or journey that all people with diabetes will take. There are many ways in which health professionals can help the person on their journey, beginning with honest, evidence-based information sharing so that they start their journey with an appropriate understanding of their condition, its causes and their treatment options.

Recognising and acknowledging the person's emotional reactions to living with diabetes is important so that they do not feel alone in their efforts to manage this unrelenting condition. Finally, diabetes is a journey that few make in isolation, so it is important to acknowledge the role of the family and society as a whole in supporting or sabotaging self-care efforts. Many people face challenges arising from over-involved family members or perceived social stigma. The journey may be unclear and the path littered with obstacles but, with the support of a trusted health professional, the individual will make their unique journey with diabetes.

Reflective questions

Reflection is a key part of the person with diabetes' journey: it is equally important for health professionals to reflect on their journey as a health professional and educator. The following are some questions you might like to reflect on. It sometimes helps if you think about a person with diabetes you educated recently and felt you did not do the job as well as you would like to.

- Select three new things you learned from reading this chapter and reflect on how you will incorporate them into your practice.
- What skills do you have to initiate a conversation about diabetes-related distress and depression?
- What skills do you need to develop to manage such a conversation next time?
- If you have diabetes, how can you focus on and listen to the individual's story, and not your own diabetes story?
- Is disclosing your diabetes to the person you are educating during a consultation/helpful?
- If so in what circumstances is it useful?
- How should it be done?
- What are the advantages and disadvantages of disclosing your diabetes?

References

Adams S, Pill R, Jones A (1997) Medication, chronic illness and identity: the perspective of people with asthma. *Social Science & Medicine* 45(2): 189–201.

Ali S, Stone MA, Peters JL, Davies MJ, Khunti K (2006) The prevalence of co-morbid depression in adults with Type 2 diabetes: a systematic review and meta-analysis. *Diabetic Medicine* 23(11): 1165–1173.

Anderson BJ, Miller JP, Auslander WF, Santiago JV (1981) Family characteristics of diabetic adolescents: relationship to metabolic control. *Diabetes Care* 4: 586–593.

Anderson, BJ, Brackett J, Ho J, Laffel L (1999) An office-based intervention to maintain parent-adolescent teamwork in diabetes management: impact on parent involvement, family conflict, and subsequent glycemic control. *Diabetes Care* 22: 713–721.

Asimakopoulou K, Skinner TC, Spimpolo J, Marsh S, Fox C (2008) Unrealistic pessimism about risk of coronary heart disease and stroke in patients with type 2 diabetes. *Patient Education and Counseling* 71(1): 95–101.

Barnard KD, Skinner TC, Peveler R (2006) The prevalence of co-morbid depression in adults with Type 2 diabetes: a systematic review and meta-analysis. *Diabetic Medicine* 23(4): 445–448.

Brar R (2005) Investigating non-compliance with treatment in people with type 2 diabetes. *Diabetes Update* Autumn: 35–38.

Brod M, Kongsø JH, Lessard S, Christensen TL (2009) Psychological insulin resistance: patient beliefs and implications for diabetes management. *Quality of Life Research* 18(1): 23–32.

Buckloh LM, Lochrie AS, Antal H, Milkes A, Canas JA, Hutchinson S, Wysocki T (2008) Diabetes complications in youth: qualitative analysis of parents' perspectives of family learning and knowledge. *Diabetes Care* 31(8): 1516–1520.

Cerkoney KAB, Hart LK (1980) The relationship between the health belief model and compliance of persons with diabetes mellitus. *Diabetes Care* 3(5): 594–598.

Chesla CA, Fisher L, Skaff MM, Mullan JT, Gilliss CL, Kanter R (2003) Family predictors of disease management over one year in Latino and European American patients with type 2 diabetes. *Family Process* 42(3): 375–390.

Ciechanowski PS, Katon WJ, Russo JE (2000) Depression and diabetes: impact of depressive symptoms on adherence, function and costs. *Archives of Internal Medicine* 160(21): 3278–3285.

Clark M (2004) *Understanding Diabetes*. Chichester: John Wiley & Sons Ltd.

Cramer J (2004) A systematic review of adherence with medications for diabetes. *Diabetes Care* 27(5): 1218–1224.

Davies M, Dempster M, Malone A (2006) Do people with diabetes who need to talk want to talk? *Diabetic Medicine* 23(8): 917–919.

Delamater AM (2006) Improving patient adherence. *Clinical Diabetes* 24(2): 71–77.

Delamater AM, Jacobson AM, Anderson B, Cox D, Fisher L, Lustman P, Rubin R, Wysocki T (2001) Psychosocial therapies in diabetes. Report of the psychosocial therapies working group. *Diabetes Care* 24: 1286–1292.

Fisher L, Chesla CA, Bartz RJ, Gilliss C, Skaff MA, Sabogal F, Kanter RA, Lutz CP (1998) The family and type 2 diabetes: a framework for intervention. *Diabetes Educator* 24(5): 599–607.

Gillibrand R, Stevenson J (2006) The extended health belief model applied to the experience of diabetes in young people. *British Journal of Health Psychology* 11(1): 155–169.

Goenka N, Dobson L, Patel V, O'Hare P (2004) Cultural barriers to diabetes care in South Asians: arranged marriage – arranged complications? *Practical Diabetes International* 21(4): 154–156.

Gherman A, Schnur J, Montgomery G, Sassu R, Veresiu I, David D (2011) How are adherence people more likely to think? A meta-analysis of health beliefs and diabetes self-care. *Diabetes Educator* 37(3): 392–408.

Hagger MS, Orbell S (2003) A meta-analytic review of the common-sense model of illness representations. *Psychology and Health* 18(2): 141–184.

Hanson C, DeGuire MJ, Schinkel AM, Kolterman OG (1995) Empirical validation for a family-centered model of care. *Diabetes Care* 18: 1347–1356.

Karter AJ, Parker MM, Moffet HH, Ahmed AT, Ferrara A, Liu JY, Selby JV (2004) Missed appointments and poor glycemic control: an opportunity to identify high-risk diabetic patients. *Medical Care* 42(2): 110–115.

Khunti K, Skinner TC, Heller S, Carey ME, Dallosso HM, Davies MJ on behalf of the DESMOND Collaborative (2008) Biomedical, lifestyle and psychosocial characteristics of people newly diagnosed with Type 2 diabetes: baseline data from the DESMOND randomized controlled trial. *Diabetic Medicine* 25(12): 1454–1461.

Kneck A, Klang B, Fagerberg I (2011) Learning to live with illness: experiences of persons with recent diagnoses of diabetes mellitus. *Scandinavian Journal of Caring Sciences* 25(3): 558–566.

Maillet N A, Melkus GD, Spollett G (1996) Using focus groups to characterize the health beliefs and practices of black women with non-insulin-dependent diabetes. *The Diabetes Educator* 22: 39–46.

Mann DM, Ponieman D, Leventhal H, Halm EA (2009) Predictors of adherence to diabetes medications: the role of disease and medication beliefs. *Journal of Behavioral Medicine* 32(3): 278–284.

McSharry J, Moss-Morris R, Kendrick T (2011) Illness perceptions and glycaemic control in diabetes: a systematic review with meta-analysis. *Diabetic Medicine* 28(11): 1300–1310.

Mosely K, Malik-Aslam A, Speight J (2010) Overcoming barriers to diabetes care: perceived communication issues of healthcare professionals attending a pilot Diabetes UK training programme. *Diabetes Research and Clinical Practice* 87(2), e11–e14.

Parry O, Peel E, Douglas M, Lawton J (2004) Patients in waiting: a qualitative study of type 2 diabetes patients' perceptions of diagnosis. *Family Practice* 21: 131–136.

Peel E, Parry O, Douglas M, Lawton J (2004) Blood glucose self-monitoring in non-insulin-treated type 2 diabetes: a qualitative study of patients' perspectives. *British Journal of General Practice* 54(500): 183–188.

Peel E, Douglas M, Lawton J (2007) Self monitoring of blood glucose in type 2 diabetes: longitudinal qualitative study of patients' perspectives. *BMJ* 335: 493.

Peyrot M, Rubin RR, Lauritzen T, Snoek FJ, Matthews DR, Skovlund SE (2005) Psychosocial problems and barriers to improved diabetes management: results of the Cross-National Diabetes Attitudes, Wishes and Needs (DAWN) Study. *Diabetic Medicine* 22(10): 1379–1385.

Pham TK. (2004) The diabetic Vietnamese population of San Diego County: The impact of ethnic-specific factors that support and inhibit the prevalence, prevention, management and treatment of diabetes. http://www.calendow.org/reference/publications/pdf/disparities/diabetes/TCE0102-2004_The_Social_E.pdf (retrieved on 18 May 2012).

Polonsky WH, Jackson RA. (2004) What's so tough about taking insulin? Addressing the problem of psychological insulin resistance in type 2 diabetes. *Clinical Diabetes* 22: 147–150.

Pouwer F, Beekman ATF, Lubach C, Snoek FJ (2006) Nurses' recognition and registration of depression, anxiety and diabetes-specific emotional problems in outpatients with diabetes mellitus. *Patient Education and Counseling* 60(2): 235–240.

Ramachandran S, Augustine C, Viswanathan V, Ramachandran A (2005) Improving psycho-social care: the Indian experience. *Diabetes Voice* 50(1): 19–21.

Samuel-Hodge CD, Headen SW, Skelly AH, Ingram AF, Keyserling TC, Jackson EJ, Ammerman AS, Elasy TA (2000) Influences on day-to-day self-management of type 2 diabetes among African-American women: spirituality, the multi-caregiver role, and other social context factors. *Diabetes Care* 23: 928–933.

Schabert J, Browne JL, Mosely K, Speight J (submitted) Social stigma in diabetes: a growing problem for an increasing epidemic. *Diabetic Medicine*.

Schillinger D, Grumbach K, Piette J, Wang F, Osmond D, Daher C, Palacios J, Sullican GD, Bindman AB (2002) Association of health literacy with diabetes outcomes. *Journal of the American Medical Association* 288(4): 475–482.

Selden CR, Zorn M, Ratzan S, Parker RM (2000) *Current Bibliographies in Medicine: Health Literacy*. Bethesda, Maryland: National Library of Medicine.

Singh H, Cinnirella M, Bradley C (submitted) Support systems for and barriers to diabetes management in South Asians and Whites in the UK: qualitative study of patients' perspectives. *BMJ*.

Skinner TC (2004) Psychological barriers. *European Journal of Endocrinology* 151: T13–T17.

Snoek FJ, Kersch NYA, Eldrup E, Harman-Boehm I, Hermanns N, Kokoszka A, Matthews DR, McGuire BE, Pibernik-Okanovic M, Singer J, de Wit M, Skovlund SE. (2011) Monitoring of individual needs in diabetes (MIND): baseline data from the Cross-National Diabetes Attitudes, Wishes, and Needs MIND Study. *Diabetes Care* 34 (3):601–603.

Snoek FJ, Pouwer F, Welch GW, Polonsky WH (2000) Diabetes-related emotional distress in Dutch and US diabetic patients: cross-cultural validity of the problem areas in diabetes scale. *Diabetes Care* 23(9): 1305–1309.

Solowiejczyk J (2004) The family approach to diabetes management: theory into practice toward the development of a new paradigm. *Diabetes Spectrum* 17(1): 31–36.

Stone M, Pound E, Pancholi A, Farooqi A, Khunti K (2005) Empowering patients with diabetes: a qualitative primary care study focusing on South Asians in Leicetser, UK. *Family Practice* 22(6): 647–652.

Telford K, Kralik D, Koch T (2006) Acceptance and denial: implications for people adapting to chronic illness: literature review. *Journal of Advanced Nursing* 55(4): 457–64.

von Wartburg L (2007) *Type 1 Pop Star, Nick Jonas Tells His Story*. http://www.diabeteshealth.com/read/2007/04/26/5150/type-1-pop-star-nick-jonas-tells-his-story (downloaded 30 Dec 2011).

Weinger K, McMurrich SJ, Yi JP, Lin S, Rodriguez M (2005) Psychological characteristics of frequent short-notice cancellers of diabetes medical and education appointments. *Diabetes Care* 28(7): 1791–1793.

Welch G, Rose G, Ernst D (2006) Motivational interviewing and diabetes: What is it, how is it used, and does it work? *Diabetes Spectrum* 19(1): 5–11.

Wen LK, Shepherd MD, Parchman ML (2004) Family support, diet, and exercise among older Mexican Americans with type 2 diabetes. *The Diabetes Educator* 30(6): 980–993.

Wing RR, Goldstein MG, Acton KJ, Birch LL, Jakicic JM, Sallis JF, Smith-West D, Jeffery RW, Surwit RS (2001) Behavioural science research in diabetes: lifestyle changes related to obesity, eating behaviour, and physical activity. *Diabetes Care* 24(1): 117–123.

3 Teaching and Learning: The Art and Science of Making Connections

Trisha Dunning AM

Deakin University and Barwon Health, Geelong, Victoria, Australia

> *Oh, Merlin,* he cried [young King Arthur] *Please come too.*
>
> *For this once* said a large solemn tench [Merlin] beside his ear,
> *I will come. But in future you will have to go by yourself.*
> *Education is experience, and the essence of experience is self-reliance.*
> White (1958, p. 41)

Introduction

It is impossible to encompass the huge body of information about teaching and learning in one chapter. Thus, Chapter 3 provides a broad overview of the field. There is no best way to teach, but there is increasing recognition that it is important to help people build connections and make meaning from what they learn, rather than merely completing tasks. Creating meaning involves developing collaborative partnerships and engaging learners (see Chapter 5).

Learning is not necessarily an outcome of teaching and many people, even well-educated people, do not understand as much as others think they do. People may be able to repeat what they were told or read, but questioning shows they do not really understand the information, or their understanding is incorrect.

Thus, educators must focus on the quality of understanding rather than the ability to regurgitate information. For example, people's 'knowledge' scores may improve after a 'diabetes education programme' but their understanding may stay the same or decline, depending on the effectiveness of the teaching and the person's ability to lay down new neural pathways that connect new information to existing information.

Diabetes Education: Art, Science and Evidence, First Edition. Edited by Trisha Dunning AM.
© 2013 John Wiley & Sons, Ltd. Published 2013 by John Wiley & Sons, Ltd.

People have to construct their own meaning from the information they receive (turn information into knowledge) by establishing permanent neural pathways and connections in the brain. If the information is not used frequently, the connections become less well established, which is why 'refresher programmes' and repeating information are important teaching strategies, and why continuing professional development is essential for health professionals.

The information in this chapter is relevant to educating people with diabetes, health professionals (HP) and educating the self. It is also applicable to individual, group and online teaching, although there are differences between the three modes.

Purpose of diabetes education

The overall purpose of diabetes education is to help people with diabetes/ family members/carers to:

- Establish a therapeutic relationship between the educator and learner(s).
- Acquire, retain and be able to use relevant information.
- Make connections between new information and existing knowledge.
- Develop problem-solving skills.
- Understand the importance of self-care to health, well-being and quality of life.
- Achieve the skills and establish behaviours and attitudes needed to self-care.
- Provide appropriate support and make appropriate referrals.

An underlying assumption is that the educator has the relevant education and assessment, teaching, clinical and helping skills, and adopts a person-centred rather than a problem-centred approach.

Principles of learning and teaching

Principles of learning were developed to support educators to work with learners. The principles focus on the educator's ability to create and maintain an environment conducive to learning. Importantly, the principles are also relevant to the educator's learning. Principles are statements about the quality of learning and the teaching methods likely to create learning environments (see Table 3.1). The principles should be considered in conjunction with the educator's teaching philosophy (see Chapter 5).

Principles were designed to be interpreted in particular learning contexts and to stimulate reflection and conversations about teaching pedagogies.

Table 3.1 **Principles of learning.**

Principle	Application to diabetes educator role
Careful planning, commitment to and resources for diabetes education are essential within busy clinical environments	Education leadership and management Advocate with and for people with diabetes Ensure the environment is as learner friendly as possible
Educators are responsible for their own learning and continuing professional development	Initial training and continued professional development Seek mentors Participate in communities of learning
Educators help each other learn and develop their pedagogies through formal education programmes, mentorship and communities of learning	Participate in communities of learning locally and internationally, e.g. IDF D-net Provide mentorship Publish and present at conferences and other learning forums
Research engagement is important to evidence-based practice, the quality of teaching, education programmes and clinical and education outcomes	Engage in research at the level of knowledge and skill Practice in an evidence-based care climate: at least must be able to critique and understand research publications Implement research findings Undertake and publish research Evaluate self and diabetes services using valid tools and processes
New understanding flows from research and reflection in and on practice	Reflection in and on practice (Chapter 5)
Educators need to collaborate with other educators to stimulate and support innovation, enhance and share their knowledge and contribute to the profession	Promote interdisciplinary team care and actively participate in team care
Educators must be willing to question existing practices and make relevant changes but change should be evolutionary rather than revolutionary	Ask good questions and higher order thinking are correlated. Educators must value and encourage people's questions
Educators need to take risks and support colleagues' risk-taking	Trying new teaching strategies such as those described in Chapter 7

Note: There are important outcomes of effective pedagogy that standard test measures do not assess. Educators often measure metabolic parameters, before and after knowledge scores. But these measures may not actually reflect *learning*. Likewise, they may only be surrogate markers for the educator's effectiveness.

Principles are not standards or curriculum statements: however, they can be used to develop curricula and standards. Importantly, principles focus on what educators should do, and are based on behavioural and learning theories.

Pedagogy encompasses ways of working with learners. Principles can help educators explore their pedagogy through reflection and discussion with other educators, which also helps bring tacit knowledge into the open for others to discuss and learn from (Polyani 1966, 1969). However, the thinking and behaviour that informs educator's pedagogy is complex and personal. In addition, teaching strategies that are effective for one educator may not be as effective for others with different levels of experience, beliefs, confidence and behaviours.

Learning theory

Learning is a process that encompasses cognitive, emotional, experiential and environmental influences people use to acquire, enhance or change knowledge, skills, values or world views (Illeris 2004). Learning theories attempt to explain what happens when learning occurs and provide educators with the vocabulary and a conceptual framework for interpreting the learning they observe and suggest teaching strategies to enhance learning (Hill 2002).

Learning theories fall into three main philosophical frameworks:

1. **Behaviourism**: primarily developed by Skinner (1954) but encompasses Thorndike, Tolman, Guthrie and Hull's work. Behaviour theories are based on three underlying assumptions:
   a. Learning results in behaviour change through conditioning.
   b. Environment shapes behaviour.
   c. The principles of contiguity and reinforcement are central to explaining the learning process.
2. **Cognitivism**: Bode (1929), a gestalt psychologist, criticised behaviourist theories as being too dependent on overt behaviour to explain learning. Gestalt theorists believed the memory system actively processes and organises information, and prior knowledge affects learning. That is, cognitive theories look beyond behaviour to explain learning and the control the learner has over the learning process. Several cognitive theories emerged between the 1970s and the 1990s and others continue to emerge as the understanding of brain functions increases. Educators using a cognitive approach regard learning as an internal mental process requiring insight, information processing, memory and perception, and design education strategies to enhance existing knowledge and skills.
3. **Constructivism**: based on Piaget, Bruner Vygotsky and Deweys' learning theories. These theorists viewed learning as a process in which the learner builds on current and past experience: 'constructing knowledge from one's own experiences'. Therefore, learning is personal. The educator helps 'bring the learner to the threshold of his own mind' (Gibran 2008). Knowledge is constructed in social contexts (social constructivism). Educators can help the learner explore social issues relevant to them to discover meaning and construct knowledge

as distinct from acquiring information: for example, self-directed, transformational and experiential learning, situated cognition and reflective practice.

Other less formal and post-modern learning theories also exist, for example, restructuring knowledge (Marzano 1991). Marzano maintained new knowledge could not be told to learners. The educator must challenge a learner's current knowledge so the learner can adjust their ideas in the light of the new information. Transformational learning involves using discourse to critically examine and reflect on habits and beliefs and seek alternative explanations. Transformational learning is more likely to lead to self-knowledge and responsible thinking (Mezirow 1991).

Educational Neuroscience or Neuroeducation theories are emerging (Radin 2009; Wolf 2010). These theories connect information about how the brain processes and stores information with education strategies, for example, conditions that enhance knowledge acquisition, storage and recall. Radin (2009) suggested the art and science of teaching accelerated after former US President GH Bush declared the 1990s 'The Decade of the Brain'.

Brain research will influence diabetes education theory and practice in the future, for example the way we educate people with learning disabilities and the ability to individualise teaching to education effectiveness.

Laws of learning

In addition to principles of teaching and learning, 'laws of learning' provide insight into how people learn. The basic laws are: readiness, exercise, effect primacy, recency, intensity and freedom (Table 3.2).

Knowledge

There is no single agreed definition of 'knowledge'. Generally, knowledge refers to expertise and the skills a person acquires through experience and/or education. But it also refers to enlightenment and cognition (Macquarie Dictionary Online 2010). Significantly, for diabetes educators:

Real knowledge is to know the extent of one's ignorance.

(Confucius 551–479 BC)

Many educators assume giving people with diabetes information is 'giving them knowledge'. However, acquiring knowledge is a complex cognitive process involving perception, learning, communication, association, reasoning

Table 3.2 **Laws of learning.**

'Law'	Implication for diabetes education
Readiness	People are more likely to learn when they are physically, mentally and emotionally ready to learn
	Factors that could affect people with diabetes' readiness to learn are age, health status, feelings about the diagnosis
Exercise/practice	If information and skills are repeated, they are easier to remember and people are more likely to retain information
	Politicians are experts at repeating information throughout speeches
	Practice must be meaningful to the individual and should be followed by positive feedback
Effect	Emotional reactions of learners directly affect learning and are related to motivation
	Learning is enhanced when it is pleasurable and satisfying. People with diabetes should leave every learning experience feeling positive
Primacy	Information learned first creates a strong impression and is difficult to erase
	The first education encounter for people with diabetes should provide accurate information in a logical stepwise manner ensuring the individual learns the preceding step before progressing to the next step
Recency	The most recently learned information/skills are more likely to be remembered
	For example, it might be a long time before an individual needs to implement 'sick day care' and they may forget key self-care activities and information
	Thus, such information could be part of an annual education review
Intensity	A clear, dramatic, exciting, positive learning experience is more likely to engender learning. People learn more from real-life situations than abstract or simulated situations
	Educators can use the individual's blood glucose tests to help the individual determine the effect of food, exercise and medicines
	Use creative teaching methods and involve at least two senses
Freedom	Things learned freely are learned best and are more likely to lead to personal growth
	Educators could involve people with diabetes in decisions about what they want to learn and the order they want to learn it in

and reflection. Thus, the individual needs to process the information and construct neural pathways and connections before information becomes part of his or her knowledge base.

Knowledge cannot be transferred directly from one person to another because of the way information is encoded and handled in the neural pathways in the brain that process information, make connections and lay down memories. Information can be transferred in many ways, especially via writing, technology and spoken and body language. Educators need to realise that incorrect information can be and is transferred and needs to be unlearned.

There are various types of knowledge. Broadly, knowledge is classified as procedural (learning tasks) and declarative (knowledge in store). In addition, knowledge is classified as:

- Spatial knowledge: which is specific to a particular situation. Learning from experience (experiential learning) creates situational knowledge.
- Experiential knowledge (*a posteriori*) gained through experience that was not there before (*a priori*).
- Partial knowledge: it is almost impossible to have complete knowledge about anything. Thus, most people have partial knowledge, which they use to solve problems and understand issues, often by sourcing other information.
- Tacit knowledge: is understood but is unspoken and implicit. People often know more than they can articulate in words. Importantly, although the individual may not be able to articulate tacit knowledge, they use such knowledge to make sense of their world.
- Scientific knowledge: which continues to contribute to the empirical basis of diabetes education and evidence-based care. Scientific knowledge is acquired by conducting research, reading about research and using inductive and deductive processes to understand research findings and apply them to diabetes education.
- Unconscious knowledge or intuition: A great deal of information processing occurs in an automatic non-conscious process that influences insight, creativity and decisions (Myers 2007; Kahneman 2011). Intuition bypasses the thinking part of the brain (cortex) and is often emotionally charged. It influences insight, creativity and prejudices 'my gut feeling tells me …'. Kahneman referred to system 1 (fast track) or intuition, which requires little energy, and system 2 (slow track) the conscious mind that employs deliberate, rational thought and requires a great deal of energy. Intuitive responses mean people form an opinion about other people in 4–6 seconds (see Chapter 5).

Health professionals (HPs) regularly us intuition, for example experienced HPs often follow mental short cuts (heuristics) when making clinical and education decisions. Many decisions are based on experiential and tacit knowledge and pattern recognition. Less-experienced HPs are more likely to follow guidelines. Intuition can lead to costly errors.

Nudging

Children and adults are influenced by small changes in context (Thaler and Sunstein 2009) and small, seemingly insignificant things, can have a significant effect on behaviour. Diabetes educators need to assume everything matters and make choices about education most likely to be beneficial: it is almost impossible to design the 'perfect education programme'.

'Nudging' aims to induce people to change behaviour without necessarily banning activities. Nudging might be a useful strategy for diabetes education, but research is needed. Nudging is based on the theory that people tend to maintain the status quo but can be 'nudged' to change. Nudges, in diabetes education could include goal incentives (negotiated with the individual) and positive feedback. Economic incentives and other forms of 'bribery' are not ethical.

Interestingly, a BBC health news report of 19 July 2011 suggested 'nudging is not enough to change lifestyles' and that change will only be possible if the Government is prepared to legislate. However, legislation might be at odds with nudge theory of not banning things.

Learning and the brain

The brain consists of millions of neurons capable of connecting with each other via dendrites. Learning occurs when a connection is made. Table 3.3 shows the parts of the brain where specific learning activities occur. Neurons communicate electronically and chemically to send and receive information. Repeated stimulation enables the connection to become permanent, if the neural pathways are used frequently. Neural pathways/connections do not disappear: they become less established with disuse, but can be reactivated when needed.

Table 3.3 **There are specific sites in the brain where particular learning activities occur.**

Left hemisphere: logical and rational	Right hemisphere: creative, intuitive
• Processes information in a logical sequential way in a stepwise manner • Processes the words and sentences used in speech	• Deals with information in a random, holistic way by processing pieces of information that are significant rather than in the order they arrive • Responds to emotive stimuli • Makes sense of the way the information was said, e.g. accent, speech clarity and intonation
Types of learning activities that stimulate the left hemisphere are: • Describing something • Learning key words • Changing written information • Writing a description	To connect to the right hemisphere use: • Drawings, diagrams, flow charts • Poetry, mnemonics, colours • Pictures, mind maps, flow charts • Visualisation

Source: Wright (2006).
Note: The neocortex is the central site for learning and is divided into two hemispheres, which work in different ways. Balanced teaching should include a range of activities that stimulate and connect both sides of the brain because both are important.

When people learn new information, the new neural pathway has to connect to existing pathways and other neurons for meaning to be made. Adults have many existing neural connections but children need first-hand experience because they do not have existing connections. The connections improve as they are used through chemical coatings on the transmitting end of the neuron that makes the connection permanent (myelination). Most of the myelination process occurs before age 16.

Encouraging children to use higher order thinking skills, for example, forming opinions about things/issues and then explaining them and evaluating or sorting information, helps make neuronal pathways permanent. Memories are a databank of knowledge and ideas in the brain. People remember things more efficiently if the new information can be connected to information stored in the databank. Engaging at least two senses facilitates learning by enhancing neural connections and making them permanent. Repetition also helps build neural pathways and connections.

Effective learning often requires more than making multiple connections between new and old information. Often people need to restructure their thinking and change established connections among the things they already know and/or discard outdated, often long-held beliefs. If rethinking and restructuring do not take place, new information can be distorted to fit existing beliefs, or discarded. People with diabetes and educators come to an education session with their own ideas, some correct, some not.

If the educator ignores or dismisses an individual's misconceptions, their original beliefs are likely to remain, even when they give correct answers to questions during the education session. Contradicting the individual is unlikely to successfully change their beliefs: the educator needs to use creative ways to help the individual examine their beliefs and accept new information.

Memory

The hippocampus and the amygdala (the emotion centre) are involved in creating memories. There are different kinds of memory: ability to recall facts, personal experiences and physical skills, and each has its own properties. Importantly, memory is distinct from intellectual ability and perception (Koch 2010).

What makes things memorable? Why do people remember some things and not others? Why are some things indelibly imprinted in memory and others vanish like champagne bubbles? Many factors determine what people remember including how much attention the individual pays to the experience, how new and interesting the experience is, and the kinds and strength of the emotions evoked. Memories and their accompanying emotions are laid down together.

Recent research suggests memory consolidation occurs through several processes that stabilise (store) a memory trace once it is acquired. Memory consolidation consists of three main processes:

- Synaptic consolidation, which occurs within the first few minutes to hours of memory encoding or learning. Synaptic memories last for approximately 24 hours although there are some exceptions. It is achieved faster than other types of memory consolidation. Distributing learning over 24 hours can enhance synaptic memory consolidation.
- System consolidation, which is a reorganisation process where memories from the hippocampus are moved to the neocortex for more permanent storage. System consolidation is a slow dynamic process that can take one to two decades.
- Reconsolidation, which occurs when previously consolidated memories are recalled and actively consolidated.

Interestingly, forgetting appears to help the brain conserve energy and improve the efficiency of short-term (working) memory and the ability to recall important details. When people concentrate on remembering things, they put in less neural effort if they forget/ignore irrelevant things. As memories age the frontal, temporal and parietal lobes take on the role of recalling memories, and the hippocampus becomes less essential as the cortical brain regions become connected closely enough for the memory to be stable (Squire et al. 2007).

Keeping the brain fit: brain training

Food and oxygen are essential to all body functions including brain function. Inadequate diet leads to 'mental fog' and lack of essential nutrients affect cognitive functions such as concentration, learning, memory and decision-making (Kiefer 2007).

Cognitive function is optimal when blood glucose is stable and within the normal range. The brain depends on a constant supply of circulating glucose because it cannot store energy: it uses 20% of the available metabolic fuel. Hyperglycaemia and hypoglycaemia inhibit mental functioning and decision-making and affect memory and learning (Cox et al. 2000). In addition, rising blood glucose in older people, with and without diabetes, has been linked to 'senior moments' and impaired function in the dentate gyrus in the hippocampus (Swaminathan 2009). This finding highlights the importance of diabetes prevention and early detection strategies and normalising blood glucose.

Iron is essential for mental clarity because it is the basis for haemoglobin in red blood cells, which transports oxygen to cells. Essential amino acids and fatty acids are crucial to support brain function.

Brain training: mind-body fitness

The fact the brain needs exercise to maintain and improve function and be able to complete challenging and stimulating activities is not new information, for example:

> *It is exercise alone that supports the spirits and keeps the mind in vigor.*
> (Cicero 106–43 bc)

Likewise, John Adams, former US President, said:

> *Old minds are like old horses: you must exercise them if you wish to keep them in working order.*

Cicero and Adam's observations appear to be partly true. Modern technology such as MRI, PET scans used in recent research show physical activity is crucial to physical and mental well-being: 'if you don't use it you lose it' (Hertzog et al. 2009). Cognition and mental functioning is enhanced by:

- Participating in activities that require thinking
- Undertaking regular physical activity
- Social engagement
- Having a positive attitude, which also enhances immunity.

The extent to which an individual engages in these activities influences cognitive functioning in older age. Older brains are able to change and 'old dogs can learn new tricks', although it may take longer to learn and older people generally do not achieve the same level of expertise they might have achieved when they were younger. The effects are likely to be long lasting.

In addition to specific memory training strategies, training people to manage thinking skills and executive functioning (strategic planning, control over what they attend to, how they manage the mind in the process) is also important, because these skills have a broader effect on cognitive functioning (Li et al. 2008; Hertzog et al. 2009). Although activities such as reading help, physical fitness that improves cardiovascular fitness and aerobic exercise are important, and if undertaken regularly in mid-life, they reduce the risk of dementia in later life.

Many 'brain gym' programmes are available but they do not all have robust evidence to support their claims and some may not improve executive functioning. Companies are being established that offer 'personalised online boot camps' to 'enhance your core ability to learn and improve your brain's health and wellbeing' (Ferguson 2011; www.eliteminds.com.au).

Some of these programmes enhance people's ability to perform tasks they are already performing more efficiently rather than boosting memory and cognition in a broad way. Peter Snyder, from the Neurosciences at Centre Brown University reviewed several brain training reports and concluded that many are not rigorous enough to support their claims. However, some programmes appear to improve a range of brain functions and bolster working memory and processing speed (Mossman 2009).

More rigorous research is required: despite the promise of brain gyms 'the best memory enhancer is physical exercise'.

Sleep: vital for learning and memory

Quintillian noted: *'the interval of a single night will greatly increase the strength of memory ... the power of recollection undergoes a process of ripening and maturing during the time which intervenes'.*

Or, as my grandmother used to say, 'sleep on it'. Sleep is important to consolidate motor skills (procedural memory) and declarative memory but not in the same way. Insight and clarity increase after sleep (Stickgold and Ellenbogen 2008). During sleep the brain:

- Appears to stop processing incoming sensory signals and information.
- Processes the day's information by sorting through recent memories, and stabilising and filing them.
- Makes memories resistant to interference from other information, which allows memories to be recalled more effectively the next day.
- Sifts through newly formed memories, probably identifying what to keep, and selectively maintaining or enhancing these memories.
- Saves important emotional elements of situations and discards less relevant background information.
- Analyses collections of memories to determine relationships among them and perhaps even find meaning in the information acquired.

Thus, adequate sleep appears to be important. Experts recommend 8 hours but individual differences need to be considered.

His brain, her brain

Not surprisingly, research also shows male and female brains differ structurally, chemically and functionally, despite other similarities (Cahill 2005). Thus, gender influences many areas of cognition and behaviour including memory, emotion, vision, hearing, processing faces and the brain's response to stress hormones. Some key differences are:

- Response to stress and remembering stressful experiences.
- Males navigate spatially, compared to females who navigate by remembering landmarks.
- Reaction to learning experiences.
- Lay down memories of emotion-laden incidents (Hines 2004).

Although some of this work is based on animal models, it suggests men and women with diabetes may learn differently and require different teaching strategies and language.

Brain research holds significant promise for the future given the increasing age of the population in many countries and the increasing prevalence of diabetes in older people.

Technology

The expanding use of technology is shaping neural processing and brain evolution (Small and Vorgan 2008) (see Chapter 12). Undertaking Internet searchers for an hour a day changes the way the brain processes information: strengthens new neural pathways and weakens old ones. Research suggests the constant barrage of e-information is stimulating and sharpens cognitive and discriminatory skills, but it is also draining.

Digital technology also influences how we think, feel and behave, and communicate. As the brain evolves and the focus shifts towards new technological skills, social skills such as reading body language or interpreting the emotional context may decline. Significantly, a lot of the exposure to technology is passive (watching TV or listening to iPods). In addition, monitoring Facebook and emails creates continuous partial attention (CPA) or distracted mental state, which is a heightened state of stress, which detracts from the time needed to reflect, contemplate and make thoughtful decisions.

Once people become accustomed to CPA they get 'high' on the perpetual connectivity because it boosts ego and self-worth. Research suggests the sense of self-worth protects the hippocampus, which allows people to learn and remember new information. However, CPA eventually causes brain strain and leads to more frequent errors, fatigue, irritability and distraction (digital fog) (Small and Vorgan 2008).

Technology itself does not guarantee learning, but it might help the educator create the conditions in which learning can occur (Driscoll 2002). Thus, it is important to use technology appropriately in diabetes education (see Chapter12), for example:

- Learning occurs in context, therefore, young children might lack knowledge but they can to reason. Computer simulations and games can offer appropriate scenarios to supply context.
- Learning is active: Learners learn more when they are mentally and emotionally involved in learning activities. Technology can enable learners to manipulate information and participate in group e-learning and problem-solving activities. Research focus groups are sometimes conducted online.
- Learning is social: As stated, technology can be isolating, unlike other programmes such as the Computer-Supported Intentional Learning Environment (CSILE) (Scardamalia and Bereiter 1994), which is a net-worked multimedia environment that enables people to collaborate about learning activities. Participants read and respond to notes and build a communal database.
- Learning is reflective: People with diabetes and educators should reflect on their learning and its outcomes. Computer programmes that include 'reflective journals' and feedback can be used.

Psychological and social research has significantly influenced teaching and learning principles, theories and laws. Table 3.4 provides an overview (but not an exhaustive list) of some psychological theories that can be applied to diabetes education.

Helping people learn: proactive strategies are more effective

Some suggestions for helping people learn are shown in Table 3.5. Many other suggestions are distributed throughout the book. Good creative writing requires the author 'to show not tell'; effective education requires the educator to show *and* tell as the following anecdote illustrates:

I just wanted to say I really enjoyed your presentation last night.

Thank you. I appreciate the feedback. It is always difficult knowing what to say at graduation ceremonies.

I went to a lecture about how to use PowerPoint to get your point across. The teacher said to use bullets and not have too much writing on the slide. He said use lots of pictures: he didn't do that in his PowerPoint, but you did. When he spoke about it I couldn't see how pictures would work, and he didn't show us. Now I know from your talk. He told us but he didn't show us. You showed and told but left space for the audience to form their own opinions.

I am pleased you enjoyed the presentation.

I really did. But you have to choose the pictures carefully, don't you? The audience has to be able to relate to the picture and understand the context.

Table 3.4 Overview of some of the psychological (behaviour) theories that influenced diabetes education; the theories are not presented in any order.

Theorist	Key message
Robert Bolton	Described 'people skills' that could help educators enhance communication skills and ability to establish relationships by focusing on listening, connecting and engaging
Edward de Bono	Effective thinking can improve creativity and problem-solving, generate alternatives and think about thinking
Nathaniel Branded	Deep needs can only come from within and get stronger the more they are developed. Educators can reflect and help people with diabetes reflect on their needs
Louann Brizendine	Men and women see the world differently Educators might need to consider gender-specific education strategies
Mihaly Csikszentmihaly	Creativity can only emerge once a person masters their work domain. Creativity can help people change the way they see, understand and appreciate things. Creativity can add fun and interest to education and enhance the learning environment. For example making up rhymes with children
Milton Erickson	The unconscious mind can provide wise solutions. Erickson used 'teaching tales' based on anecdotes from his life to establish rapport, enabled people to glean messages from the anecdotes and use show as well as tell to engage people in learning
Victor Frankyl	People can be transformed if they accept suffering (wound) or fate and can be transformed and achieve great things Facing unchangeable fate with great courage
Howard Gardner	Theory of multiple intelligences that questioned using single IQ test. The theory challenged teaching strategies and gave rise to various descriptions of learning styles such as Kolb (1984), Honey and Mumford (1986) and Hopson and Scally (1986)
Daniel Goleman	Emotional intelligence that suggests the individual's characteristics, personality, a skills and drive for exceptional performance motivates people to become self-regulated, self-aware and motivated and able to see the big picture Later social intelligence theories
William James	Psychology is the science of mental life. Everybody sees the world differently and personal consciousness is not the same from day-to-day
Abraham Maslow	Hierarchy of needs theory. People can only be fulfilled and self-actualised when basic needs are met Applied to education, the world is changing and aiming for the basics may no longer be acceptable. Educators have a responsibility to strive for excellence for themselves and help people with diabetes achieve the best they can
Ivan Pavlov	People may be less autonomous than they think. For example, educators might not salivate when a bell rings (unless it is a fire bell) but automatically refer to guidelines or tick boxes on an assessment log, that is, we are trained to our work culture

(Continued)

Table 3.4 *(continued)*

Theorist	Key message
B.F. Skinner	Learning is a function of change in overt behaviour as a result of a stimulus Reinforcement is important to strengthen the response. Reinforcers can be anything relevant to the individual, e.g. praise (as long as the reinforcer is ethical)
Carl Rogers	A genuine relationship or interaction is one where individuals feel comfortable to be themselves and can see each other's potential For diabetes education the individual guides the process, care should be person-centred, listening is essential It is necessary to heal the self because 'life is a flowing process of becoming'
Edward Deci	Self-determination theory, another way of considering locus of control: Internal, self-directed and motivated External, under other control, e.g. HP, fate, family, diabetes Suggest educators must consider satisfying intrinsic effects: Competence, succeeding Relatedness, connecting with others Autonomy, being in control
Andrew Perrin/Ziva Kunda	Motivated reasoning, which concerns starting with a conclusion one hopes to reach and selectively evaluating evidence/information to achieve the desire and discarding the rest, i.e. find ways to support preconceived ideas Educators need to recognise motivated reasoning in themselves and people with diabetes and use strategies to build confidence, promote questioning Motivated reasoning can lead to inappropriate decisions and self-care and education practices

Note: The information was derived from a number of sources, primarily Butler-Burdon (2007) Deci and Ryan (1985) and Kunda (1990).
Seven out of ten leading causes of death are linked to behaviour (Harris and Lustman 1998).

Another important issue is to try to ensure information and messages are consistent among HPs.

> *Listen to them! They're all playing different tunes!*
> Well, *for 55 days they played the **same** tune.*
>
> (Fifty Five Days at Peking 1963)

Inconsistent information creates confusion, is a disincentive to learning and may cause the individual to doubt some or all HPs' knowledge and credibility. We need to play the same tune all the time—the challenge is HOW?

Table 3.5   **Teaching strategies should suit the individual or group and consider the principles and laws of learning.**

Learning	Teaching strategy
Ensure the environment is conducive to learning	Private Quiet Position seats Try to minimise interruptions Try to commence the session on time Find out what the individual expects to achieve
Be informed, flexible and use appropriate language	Develop the relevant skills and knowledge Determine the individual's story and existing knowledge Attend and be present in the encounter (Chapters 5 and 6)
Establish a relationship with the individual	Be present and connected Use congruent body language Use appropriate questions to clarify and collect information Show empathy and understanding Be mindful of signs of distress Determine goals for the session and management goals with the individual
Progress from the known to the unknown and concrete to the abstract	Find out what the person already knows and build on the information and help them connect new information to existing information Young people learn best about tangible tings they can touch, feel and smell. As they develop they learn to understand abstract concepts and reason logically People construct meaning by connecting information to existing knowledge. Educators can help people explore their existing knowledge and beliefs so they can build on or help the person change existing knowledge
People learn when they are able to practice and are actively engaged in experiential learning	For example, ask them to find information in a brochure, interpret their blood glucose patterns and/or think of a reason for the pattern and strategies for managing the issue Practice is important for tasks such as blood glucose monitoring but also for solving-problems, recognising patterns Practice is more effective if it matches the individual's goals Activities should be challenging but achievable
People require positive feedback to learn effectively	To become self-caring people with diabetes need to learn to monitor their body cues and adjust to compensate, e.g. recognise and treat a hypo. Allow the individual to express their opinions and provide feedback/suggestions at the teachable moment (an example of where they should be used) Use mistakes as learning opportunities
Learning is affected by expectations	People have ideas about what they can and cannot do/learn. This is partially related to their locus of control and views about their competence. Building confidence and praise are important
Use evidence when appropriate	People want evidence-based care but they may need help interpreting the scientific language and applying it to their unique situation

(Continued)

Table 3.5   *(continued)*

Learning	Teaching strategy
Use activities to help learners find answers for themselves	Use appropriate questions Suggest they read specific information and decide whether it is appropriate to their situation Help the individual develop problem-solving skills Use mistakes as teaching opportunities
Welcome questions, and people's stories	Questions help people learn—they usually ask a question because they want an answer Try not to put the question off until 'later' People's stories are a clue to who they are and how to help them learn and become self-caring
Use mistakes as learning opportunities	Help the individual reflect on the issue and the context surrounding it and engage in problem-solving to make relevant changes
Be creative and engage both sides of the brain	Children love stories and rhymes. Create a story about their diabetes or use existing books written for children Familiar 'nursery rhymes' were originally social commentaries, e.g. Ring a Ring of Roses referred to the plague, Mary, Mary, Quite Contrary to Queen Mary's (Bloody Mary) Catholicism

Note: We don't receive wisdom; we must discover it for ourselves after a journey that no one can take for us or spare us (Marcel Proust).

Asking the 'right' questions to encourage conversation rather than debate is an art (see Chapter 2). Use open, probing questions. Leading questions are appropriate to elicit some information. 'Good' questioning involves:

- Attending and active listening
- Paraphrasing core information: *It sounds like …*
- Reflecting feelings: *You seem unsure about …*
- Reflecting meaning: *You feel … Because … is that correct?*
- Mirroring, but not too often or you might sound like a parrot: *Use the individual's words but not their tone of voice*
- Summarising: *The issues that seem to be emerging from what you are telling me are … have I missed anything?*

Consider including fun in teaching strategies. Aristotle said 'Laughter is a bodily exercise precious to health'. Research appears to support Aristotle's belief: laughter assists people to achieve cognitive distance from stress, which is psychologically protective. Laughter also helps manage pain, and cheerfulness facilitates relationships (Bennett and Lengacher 2008). Humour needs to be culturally appropriate and used with discretion.

Summary

Teaching and learning is an interrelated process. It should be person-centred, collaborative and holistic. Turning information into knowledge is a complicated process that occurs within the brain through establishing neural pathways and connections.

> **Reflective questions**
>
> Reflection is essential to learning. It is a key part of the person with diabetes' journey and it is equally important for health professionals to reflect on their journey as carers and educators. The following statements or questions may help you reflect. It sometimes helps if you think about a recent encounter with a person with diabetes where you felt the encounter did not go as well as you would like.
>
> - Do you have a teaching pedagogy?
> - If so, how did you develop your pedagogy?
> - What new or different teaching strategies could you try?
> - Is your teaching environment conducive to learning?
> - If not, what could you do to change it?

References

BBC News: Health. (2011) Nudge is not enough to changes lifestyle—Peers, 19 July 2011. http://www.bbc.co.uk/news/health-14187802 (accessed August 2011).

Bennett M, Lengacher C. (2008) Humor and laughter may influence health. Part 3: Laughter and health outcomes. *Evidence-Based Complementary and Alternative Medicine* 6(1):37–40.

Bode B. (1929) *Conflicting Psychologies of Learning.* Boston, MA, D.C. Heath and Company.

Cahill L. (2005) His brain, her brain. *Scientific American* 292:40–43.

Cox D, Gonder-Frederick L, Julian D, Cryer P, Clarke W. (2000) Progressive hypoglycaemia's impact on driving performance, occurrence, awareness and correction. *Diabetes Care* 23:163–170.

Deci EL, Ryan RM. (1985) Self determination theory. http://www.psych.rochester.edu.SDT

Driscoll M. (2002) How people learn and what technology might have to do with it. ERIC Digest ERIC Clearinghouse on Information and Technology Syracuse, New York. http://www.ericdigests.org/2003-3/learn.htm (accessed July 2011)

Ferguson D. (2011) How long till cognitive overload causes a major Australian air disaster. www.eliteminds.com.au (accessed September 2011).

Fifty Five Days at Peking. (1963) Samuel Bronston Productions.

Gibran K. (2008) *Kahlil Gibran's the Prophet and the Art of Peace*. The. New Illustrated Edition. London, Duncan Baird Publishers, p. 99.

Harris M, Lustman P. (1998) The psychologist in diabetes Care. *Clinical Diabetes* 16:1–17.

Hertzog C, Kramer A, Wilson R, Lindenberger U. (2009) Fit body, fit mind. *Scientific American Mind* July–August:24–31.

Hill W. (2002) *Learning: A Survey of Psychological Interpretation*, 7th edn. Boston, MA, Allyn and Bacon.

Hines M. (2004). *Brain Gender*. Oxford, Oxford University Press.

Honey P. Mumford A. (1986) *Using Your Learning Styles*. Maidenhead, Peter Honey.

Hopson B, Scally M. (1986) *Lifeskills Teaching Programmes* (No. 3). Leeds, Lifeskills Associates.

Illeris K. (2004) *Three Dimension of Learning*. Malabar, Krieger Publishing.

Kahneman D. (2011) *Thinking Fast and Slow*. London, Penguin.

Kiefer I. (2007) Brain food. *Scientific American Mind* October–November:58–61.

Koch C. (2010) You must remember this. *Scientific American Mind* September–October:16–20.

Kolb D. (1984) *Experiential Learning: Experience as a Source of Learning and Development*. Englewood Cliffs, NJ, Prentice-Hall.

Kunda, Z. (1990). The case for motivated reasoning. *Psychological Bulletin* 108(3):480–498.

Li S-C, Schmiedek F, Huxhold O, Rocke C, Smith J, Lindenberger U. (2008) Working memory plasticity in old age: Practice, gain and maintenance. *Psychology and Acing* 28(4):731–742.

Macquarie Dictionary Online. (2010) Correct as is the title is the Macquarie Dictionary. www.macquariedictionary.com.au (accessed July 2011).

Marzano R. (1991) Fostering thinking across curriculum through knowledge restructuring. *Journal of Reading* 34:518–525.

Mezirow J. (1991) *Transformative Dimensions of Adult Learning*. San Francisco, CA, Jossey-Bass.

Mossman K. (2009) Brain trainers. *Scientific American Mind* April–May–June:32–35.

Myers D. (2007) The powers and perils of intuition. *Scientific American Mind* June–July:24–29.

Polyani M. (1966) *The Tacit Dimension*. London, Routledge and Kegan Paul.

Polyani M. (1969) *Personal Knowledge: Toward a Post Critical Philosophy*. London, Routledge and Kegan Paul.

Radin J. (2009) Brain compatible teaching and learning: Implications fro teacher education. *Education Horizon* 88(1):40–50.

Scardamalia M, Bereiter C. (1994) Computer support for knowledge-building environments. *Journal of Learning Sciences* 3(3):265–283.

Skinner B. (1954) The science of learning and the art of teaching. *Harvard Educational Review* 24(2):86–97.

Small G, Vorgan G. (2008) Meet your iBrain. *Scientific American Mind* October–November:43–49.

Squire L, Wixted J, Clark R. (2007) Recognition memory and the medial temporal lobe: A new perspective. *Nature Reviews Neuroscience* 8(11):872–883.

Stickgold R, Ellenbogen M. (2008) Quiet! Sleeping brain at work. *Scientific American Mind* August–September:22–27.

Swaminathan N. (2009) An end to senior moments. *Scientific American* April–May:9.

Thaler R, Sunstein C. (2009) *Nudge: Improving Decisions about Health, Wealth and Happiness*. London, Penguin.

White T. (1958) *The Once and Future King*. London, Collins.

Wolf P. (2010) *Brain Matters: Translating Research into Classroom Practice*. Alexandria, VA, ASCD.

Wright D. (2006) *Classroom Karma: Positive Teaching, Positive Behaviour, Positive Learning*. London, Davis Fulton Publishers, pp. 1–28.

4 Making Choices, Setting Goals

Timothy Skinner

Rural Clinical School, University of Tasmania, Burnie, Tasmania, Australia

> *Since the human body tends to move in the direction of its expectations,*
> *plus or minus, it is important to know that attitudes of confidence*
> *and determination are no less a part of the treatment program*
> *than medical science and technology.*
>
> Norman Cousin (1979)

Introduction

Diabetes education is probably the most common activity that occurs in diabetes centres. Yet much of the literature about diabetes education driven out of empowerment work refers to diabetes education as more art than science. *The Art of Empowerment* by Anderson (2000) is just one example of the books that focus on diabetes education and care as an art, rather than science. However, the emphasis on the art of diabetes education is only one side of the coin. There is an abundance of research with Anderson's colleagues on one side and a plethora of medical texts about diabetes pathophysiology, diagnosis and treatment on the other side. I suggest the point of the tension between these two positions is probably the space where the proponents of science and art meet, converge and have some productive conversations over a glass of red wine.

I hope this chapter will meet you at the point of convergence; but I will be talking from the science side of the fence, for no other reason than I am a psychologist trained as a scientist not an artist. One of my research passions is to inform the practice of diabetes care, education and support from a position of empiricism. Likewise, I am an inherent sceptic, which makes me do quite well at critical analysis of research, but generally makes rather inept at appraising art.

The other perspective I bring to the chapter is not scientific: it is the lens I bring as a person. I am a great believer in making these lenses explicit, in the hope that the reader, using a different lens, can see what is inherently useful in what I write, and what is just a function of the lens I am wearing at particular places in the chapter. The two lenses currently tinting my thinking share many similarities and yet appear quite disparate: the lens of Soto Zen Buddhism and the Argentine Tango. The things that unite these views are the richness obtained from simplicity, from being in the present moment and connecting with the unique expression of one's self.

The emphasis is on being fully present, whether mediating alone, or entwined in the dialogue of passionate tango. These are the key to diabetes education regardless of whether you are an artist or a scientist, or sit at the intersection of the two; high quality diabetes education means being completely present in the interaction in mind and body.

Given this preamble, which I hope has been somewhat more entertaining or informative than I usually read in text books, I plan to consider three issues that I hope will help you reflect on the way you think about and deliver diabetes education. The first reflection concerns the nature of the goals people have and how goals shape decision-making. The second concerns the implications of some recent research on people's ability to resist temptation. Third, I will draw attention to an issue of increasing interest to me, both in terms of the physiological effects and what it means for education—the impact of sleep, or lack of it.

Why don't people do what is best for them?

The first area to consider is decision-making, or as one colleague said at a recent conference, 'it is amazing how many people do stupid things'. I chose not to enter into a debate with him about this throwaway line, because it sums up one common misconception that abounds in diabetes care—people do not do what clinicians think is good for them, and make what clinicians consider to be stupid decisions. I do not subscribe to such a view. In fact, I think this mindset or attitude is actually a barrier to providing effective diabetes care and education. It is based on the premise that if people are not doing what clinicians deem the appropriate thing to do (what is best for them) there is something wrong with them.

In contrast, one of my core philosophies that underpins all my work, although sometimes I forget and appear quite arrogant and condescending, so I am told, is that every individual with intact mental faculties, which excludes people with psychosis, mental disabilities and politicians, make decisions to optimise their quality of life according to their perception of their situation.

When I put this point of view forward at workshops and seminars, I am always stunned at the controversy it causes for many people. Thus, I choose to explore or expand on part of the issue in this chapter. The issue is fundamental to helping health professionals (HPs) understand their clients, support them and provide them with the tools and information they need to make informed decisions about their diabetes.

When I say 'informed decisions', I want to be clear, that I do not mean the decision, I, or any other HP, carer, friend or politician wants the individual to make. I mean exactly what I say. The individual makes an informed decision. Clinicians often assume that if they provide people with information about their diabetes, its management and the likely consequences of different actions, people with diabetes will be empowered to make informed decisions, on the understanding that people make choices, and continue to make choices each day, as they live with their diabetes. That is not what I mean by making informed decisions.

First, we have to ask whether the way we provide information to people with diabetes is done in a way that ensures they understand the information. There is sufficient research to indicate that much of the way HPs 'inform' people about their diabetes does not facilitate understanding, or even recall. Even the information leaflets and web pages we develop are not readable by or comprehensible to the vast majority of people with diabetes, or even some HPs (Petterson et al. 1994; Harwood and Harrison 2004; Boulos 2005).

However, that is not the main point: clinicians usually think an informed decision results in the person making the dietary changes the HP wants them to make or being more physically active, or taking their medication. Actually, just making recommended changes is not necessarily informed decision-making. An informed decision is based on the person considering their understanding of diabetes, regardless of whether their understanding is erroneous or not, their understanding of other aspects of their life, and their values before they decide what to do.

Thus, an individual may know that it is 'better to eat a healthy diet' but be constrained by the cost of fresh food or their family may be unwilling to eat it, and decide to continue to buy cheaper highly processed high fat food. That is an informed choice. Therefore, an informed decision is a decision where the person acts on their understanding of the information provided to them or they source for themselves, and it means the choice can be reviewed at another time. People make decisions according to what they believe will optimise their quality of life, given their perception of their situation at the time the decision is made. Thus, in the scenario described, the individual decided to continue to eat a less healthy diet for the quality of life benefits that come from managing a demanding home environment in the way that causes the least aggravation.

The key message for HPs is to understand why some people make choices that do not seem to be designed to optimise their quality of life. Common scenarios that HPs could reflect on include:

- Why do some girls consciously choose not to inject their insulin to manipulate their weight?
- Why do some people behave in ways they know will prevent their foot ulcers from healing and could lead to an amputation?

As I strived to understand people's decision-making from a scientist's perspective, I found the writings of two American psychologists, Carver and Scheier, very informative.

Self-regulation, goals and values

Carver and Scheier (2001) suggested the key to understanding people's decision-making about everyday behaviours is to understand their values and/or goals. These goals form hierarchical structures (Figure 4.1). Everyday behaviours such as preparing food and walking the dog are referred to as 'do' goals, serving higher order goals such as being a loving partner are referred to as be goals, and possibly higher goals related to core values that people hold as images of the ideal self.

The implication of Carver and Scheier's (2001) approach to behaviour being goal-orientated, is that, to understand the behaviours individuals undertake and their decision-making, HPs need to understand what the individual's goals are, and possibly more importantly the goals the behaviours are serving. Although many goals may be common to many people, each person has a different set of goals and values. Many people are not aware of their goals, because they were adopted without conscious effort through education, socialisation and culture. In addition, many goals are shared goals, for example to be healthy, liked or rich, although the importance of each goal may be different for each individual. However, other goals are relatively uncommon, or even unique to an individual. Therefore, each person has an individual goal system, which is unique to them.

Understanding peoples' values or goals can help HPs understand why people make some of the choices they make. For example, a former female military officer I counselled struggled to lose weight, get fit and be healthy

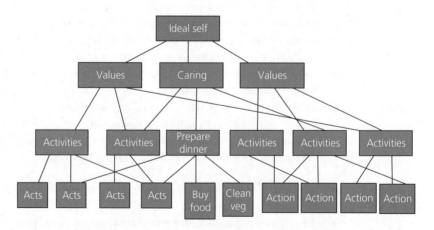

Figure 4.1 **Representation of goal hierarchies; veg = vegetables.**

and successful, because she always seemed to sabotage her own efforts. When I took time to explore the issues with her, we both began to understand that she had developed a goal to be unattractive to avoid sexual harassment.

The goal subconsciously developed over several years as she suffered unpleasant harassment in one particular military establishment. It took a great deal of effort for her to realise she had not consciously set out to make herself unattractive by being overweight. Thus, her eating and sabotaging her efforts to manage her weight made perfect sense in the context of this unconscious goal. Becoming aware of the issue enabled her to drop the goal and discontinue behaviours that serviced the goal. I am not suggesting that diabetes education should involve delving into peoples goals, but appreciating that each individual has competing sets of goals, and understanding the individual may not be aware of some goals could help HPs be less judgemental of other peoples' behaviour.

Behaviour-serving goals

If people have a set of internal goals, many of which may be competing with each other, how do they decide, consciously or otherwise, which goals have greater priority and are enacted? When I say 'decide', I am not necessarily referring to a conscious process. Many daily decisions are not consciously made, and it takes a lot of effort to bring them to awareness. For instance, I still find it exceptionally difficult to only eat one or two chocolate digestive biscuits or chocolate hob-nobs. If I have one, it takes an exceptional degree of effort of will not to eat the whole packet. I do not know why this is so, and I do not know what triggers the need to eat the whole packet of biscuits. My non-conscious mind periodically overrides my conscious goals. If other HPs are truly honest with themselves, they will be able to identify similar behaviours in themselves. Thus, it should be no great surprise that the same kind of thing happens to many people on a regular basis.

One way of understanding behaviour is to consider the goal hierarchy. Carver and Scheier (2001) argued that any specific behaviour is more likely to be enacted when it serves multiple higher order goals (Figure 4.2). Thus, behaviour B is more likely to be enacted than behaviour A, because it serves higher goals. A behaviour such as eating fruits and vegetables that only serves one goal (healthy eating) is less likely to be enacted, whereas an alternative behaviour such as walking the dog, which may serve multiple goals, for example increasing physical activity, being a responsible pet owner and managing stress, is more likely to be enacted. A second factor to consider is how well a behaviour serves its higher order goals. Thus, in Figure 4.2, behaviour B serves the middle higher goal much more effectively than the other three goals.

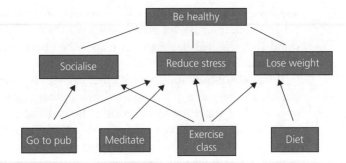

Decisions based on:
* Number of higher order goals served
* Value placed on goals
* Efficacy of actions to serve goals.

Figure 4.2   **Representation of the relationship between actions and values.**

Another issue is how important a goal is in itself at each hierarchical level. For instance, the goal of providing financial security for the family is more important for some people than exercising frequently to optimise their own health. Of course, the importance of the various goals will change as circumstances change. For example, as children complete university and start out on their careers, maintaining health may become more important than providing financial security for children.

The time urgency of goals is also likely to affect choices. For example, the fact that this chapter was well overdue to Trisha kept me indoors writing at one time rather than going outside for a long walk in the country with my dog: thus, a behaviour that serves higher important goals exceptionally well. More urgent/important goals are more likely to be enacted than a behaviour that only serves one, if any low, importance goal, poorly and in the longer term.

The ideas around goals and their hierarchies becomes richer and has implications for understanding decision-making if the differences between approach goals versus avoidance goals are considered. Avoidance goals are problematic on a number of levels. First, an avoidance goal or value, e.g. 'don't be attractive' means people never actually reach or attain the goal or its sub-goals. People can never be far enough from an avoidance goal, because they are trying to get as far away from it as possible. This also means they never get any respite from an avoidance goal because they constantly make sure they are as far away from the goal as possible.

If an individual decides to set themselves a goal to never drink again, they constantly struggle not to drink. Even if it is a time-limited goal—'I won't drink this week'—they never feel they achieve or attain the goal. They might achieve it just at the moment they fall asleep at the end of the week, but the goal is back first thing in the morning when they wake up, and the struggle begins again. This fact partly explains why abstinence goals such as to quit smoking, stop drinking or stop eating chocolate are so demanding and difficult to achieve. In addition, the problem of catastrophic failure, that is when one slip up, one cigarette, one drink, or one piece of chocolate cake, leads to dropping the goal.

If people fail once, for example take a single drag of a cigarette or eat a single piece of chocolate, their goal was not achieved for the week—they have 'failed' and might as well give up, eat the whole box of chocolates and start again next week. Thus, discrepancy-enlarging goals, or goals to avoid something such as sexual harassment, create major challenges for peoples' internal decision-making systems. Consider the lady who decided to make herself unattractive to men because of unpleasant sexual harassment and experiences. Reflect on the following questions:

- Can she ever feel unattractive enough?
- When will her weight be sufficient to convince her that she has attained or achieved her goal?

So, what lessons do these issues have for diabetes education and how to help people with diabetes? HPs must understand people's behaviours and the different goals and needs they are serving. Lack of information is rarely the main barrier to people living their lives in a way that optimises their chances of avoiding diabetes complications. Finding ways to help people understand that some of their behaviours may serve other goals and that they may not be consciously aware of these needs and goals can be helpful. In addition, helping individuals link healthy behaviours to other goals beyond just being healthy, for example losing weight can serve goals of being more active, feel less self-conscious so that they can serve multiple goals with different behaviours, might have a positive effect on their blood glucose, lipids and blood pressure and could help them lead the lives they wish as well as achieve their life goals. Importantly, helping people focus their efforts on approach goals, rather than negative and avoidance goals, may make it easier for people to achieve their goals.

This may sound like a nice theoretical explanation, but what has it got to do with educating people with diabetes? One of my goals in writing this chapter was to encourage HPs to move away from the traditional mind set of diabetes education: which to me is merely regurgitating diabetes information. I hope some of the implications of changing the traditional diabetes education process would have become evident as you read this chapter, but as the editor of the book pointed out to me, hope is not enough.

The implications of thinking about people's goals and what they want to achieve is that education will engage the person with diabetes, make them work harder to understand information and convert it into knowledge, so they are more likely to act on information when they can see how it relates to their goals. For instance, one young adult who had extremely high HbA$_{1c}$ levels and frequent hypos did not engage with the usual diabetes education patter. When he was referred to me I asked him:

'What is your goal for your diabetes?'

He answered *'for it not to interfere with my life'*.

He felt that if he ignored his diabetes and performed the self-care he needed when he thought it appropriate, his diabetes would stay in the background and not affect his life.

To engage him in further conversation, I him asked him:

'How well is your current plan working?'

He asked *'what do you mean?'* which enabled us to explore how ignoring his diabetes was working in terms of preventing diabetes from impacting on his life. We discussed how his current plan resulted in hypos, constant nagging from friends, frequent appointments at the diabetes centre, lack of energy and frustration with and about diabetes. The discussion created an opportunity to discuss some alternative ways of reaching his goals and mechanisms for evaluating different goals.

A simple way for HPs to use these techniques is to make sure the education they provide addresses the concerns of the person with diabetes. That can only be achieved by truly listening and helping the person with diabetes find the answer for themselves. In all clinical encounters, whether in a 5 min individual session or in 6 hours of group education in 1 day, a primary question to begin with is:

'What do you want to get out of the interaction to make it worth your while being here?'

It is a simple question, and immediately engages the person/people and helps ensure you address their concerns in the education session, because the information you provide is more likely to be related to their goals. You can find examples of other useful questions in Chapter 2.

Limited resources

One of the challenges people face is that, although they have multiple goals and values, they (and HPs) have limited resources with which to pursue their goals. Significantly, resources are limited in all areas of life, physical, financial, intellectual, social and emotional. Thus, people need to decide how to invest their limited resources to meet competing, different demands. Some recent research into how minds and brains function is particularly relevant to diabetes education, the concept of limited resources and people's ability to make changes in their lives. One of the key concepts is referred to as ego resiliency or impulse control. Impulse control concerns the ability to resist temptation and delay gratification. For example, when I am presented with a delicious tiramisu with short bread ice cream and chilli sugar at my local Italian restaurant, I have a choice. I can resist temptation and go home, or I can indulge!

The ability to resist temptation emerges early in people's development and is substantially different among individuals. A classic piece of research that tested young children's ability to resist temptation was to present them with a few small sweets and tell them you are about to leave the room for 5 min and if they do not eat the sweets before you return, you will give them some more sweets when you return. They can eat the sweets if they want to, but if they do so they will not get any more. Some children ate the sweets but others waited for the researcher to come back and gratefully received more. It is not surprising to note that the ability to resist temptation and delay gratification is a strong predictor of achievement in later life. It is also related to the concept of conscientiousness, which is a good predictor of longevity (Friedman et al. 1993).

Significantly, the ability to resist temptation is resource dependent. The relationship between the ability to resist temptation and achievement was demonstrated by asking individuals to perform a task that demands a high-level cognitive functioning. When the individual completes the task, they are immediately asked to complete a second, similar type of task. People's performance on the second task was much poorer than their performance on the first task, which indicates the first task depleted the individual's resources and thus their ability to complete the second task (Hagger et al. 2010).

In one set of elegant studies, Galliot and Baumeister (2007) demonstrated that if the individual is given time to recover, they can perform equally well on the second task. Further, performance seemed to be related to blood glucose levels. That is, in people without diabetes, tasks requiring the individual to resist taking an action seemed to be particularly demanding of blood glucose, dropping the blood glucose levels, although they were still within the normal range. When given time to recover, blood glucose levels return to pre-testing levels and performance is maintained. The fall in blood glucose is within in the normal range, but demonstrates how sensitive these tasks are to fluctuations in blood glucose levels.

Brain scans and ECG studies indicate these tasks rely heavily on the frontal lobes. The frontal lobes are the most recently developed parts of the human brain; thus, they are most sensitive to fluctuations in circulating blood glucose levels (Galliot and Baumeister 2007). Significantly, frontal lobe functioning is the first to be disturbed during hypoglycaemia.

Although the contention that there are individual differences in ego resiliency and people's ability to recover from these kinds of tasks may seem fatalistic, past decades show that the brain and brain function do not develop until early adulthood, then slowly decline, as was the dogma. However, recent research indicates the human brain is remarkably responsive to its environment and activities (Kramer et al. 2004). It is capable of changing its abilities, function and structure, depending on the activity the brain is asked to engage in. Thus, the brain shares similarities with the muscles; that is, both can be trained, and respond to that training to become more efficient, more responsive and stronger.

The implication of this research is that individuals can develop their brains, even in older adulthood. Therefore, with practice, individuals can become better at resisting temptation, because their brains can change and become better at doing things. This ability should not be underestimated but should be harnessed in effective diabetes education strategies. Mental activity should also be included as a core component of comprehensive diabetes care programmes. Indeed, several trials investigating whether mental activity helps prevent cognitive decline and dementia are underway (FINGER 2010).

These findings have implications for how HPs support people to make behaviour changes that will optimise their diabetes outcomes. If HPs focus on abstinence goals, we are asking people to constantly resist temptation, which will constantly deplete their mental resources, making it increasingly difficult for them to resist temptation. Further, the resources needed to achieve stop or reduce goals constantly compete with the other demands in an individual's life. If the competing goals have greater urgency for the individual, they will deplete resources necessary to work on the health behaviour stop or reduce goals. However, helping people focus on achieving positive goals will place fewer demands on their resource-limited capacity, and increase the likelihood they will achieve their goals.

One way of using this information in clinical practice is by supporting individuals to set SMART goals, or even SMARTER goals. There are a number of versions of the acronym SMART. I would like to explain my version.

SMARTER

S is for Specific, which is consistent across all the versions of the acronym I know. It means helping the person break the goal down to specific actions such as what, when, how often, how long. The more specific detail provided the better. The key is move from the vague goal 'going to being more active' to a specific goal 'I will walk for 30 min on Monday, Wednesday and Thursday as soon as I get home from work'.

M is for able to be monitored, where the focus is on how the individual will monitor how well they managed to achieve their goal. Questions to ask the individual include 'How well it is going? How many times did you manage to walk last week?'

A is for Action. Goals need to be specified in terms of the actions that are needed to achieve the goals. That is, a goal stating 'I will not do something such as not eating chocolate' will not help people as much as helping them focus on what they could do or eat. Significantly, HbA_{1c}, lipids and weight are not actions. They are the result of actions. Action goals focus on what the person will do, not the outcomes of their actions.

R is for realistic. Help people check whether they can achieve the goal. Setting a goal that an individual is unlikely to achieve is setting them up to fail, even if they set the goal themselves. Ask 'Do you think you can achieve your goal in 3 months?' You can ask them to rate the likelihood of success on a scale of one to ten. If the person scores less than seven, the goal is unrealistic and needs to be changed.

T is for time-limited. Try to move people away from the idea that the change is something they have to do and achieve for the rest of their life. Such and explanation can instantly switch people of because it is a very difficult thing to achieve. Rather, help people to focus on achieving the goal for a time-limited period. Ask people when they would like to review how well things are going.

E is for expect problems. Help people think about what things are likely to stop them from achieving their goal, then help them find solutions to the biggest barriers so they are prepared and can problem-solve more effectively when such problems arise.

R is for review and reiterate. That is, make sure you set a time to review the goal with the person and how you will do that: in person, by telephone or in a group session. After the review, it is important to reiterate the process. Review and reiterate is a continual process to support people to achieve the changes they want in their lives.

Sleep

Sleep, particularly disturbed sleep, is another factor that affects peoples' psychological resources and ability to make lifestyle changes. The recent diabetes and wider physiological literature documents the importance of a good nights sleep for optimal physical functioning (Van Cauter 2011). Short duration or disturbed sleep is predictive of obesity, increases insulin resistance and circulating levels of pro-inflammatory cytokines and reduces psychological resources (Banks and Dinges 2007; Waters and Bucks 2011). Thus, people who persistently have short or disturbed sleep are in a double bind: one is the detrimental effect on their body; the other is the impact on the psychological resources needed to enact behaviour change.

Sleep disturbance is common in people with diabetes. Many individuals with type 2 diabetes suffer from obstructive sleep apnoea (OSA), although definitive prevalence data is not available (Van Gauter 2011). Even though there is an efficacious treatment for OSA, for example constant positive airway pressure, the majority of people prescribed such treatment do not make sufficient use of it to realise the full therapeutic benefits (Lindberg et al. 2006). Depression and anxiety, also common in people with diabetes, are both associated with disturbed sleep patterns (Baran and Richert 2003). Research indicates that depression is two to three more common in people with diabetes, and, given the high prevalence of OSA, a conservative estimate suggests 30–40% of individuals with type 2 diabetes have intermittent or persistent problems with depression and/or anxiety (Ali et al. 2006).

These facts suggest that sufficient restful sleep is an important part of holistic needs and should be part of a holistic health assessment, especially when people are struggling to make lifestyle changes. The impact of sleep disturbances on people's ability to make changes should not be underestimated. Likewise, many antidepressants and sedatives used continuously for extensive periods actually lead to disturbed sleep – read the medicine information leaflets. Specialist sleep assessment and management services should be considered for people with diabetes with disturbed sleep. However, helping the individual adopt basic sleep principles can have a substantial impact on their sleep pattern, although they can take a couple of weeks to have an effect.

Summary

Diabetes management and education is very important. The way information is provided influences people's behaviours and thus outcomes. The way information is presented can increase or reduce the individual's ability to make informed decisions about their treatment and influences whether they actively participate in the discussion. Educators need to understand how people make decisions and the philosophy and science that underpins people's goals and the behaviours they serve, and conduct meaningful conversations to achieve SMARTER goals.

Reflective questions

Reflection is a key part of the journey of the person with diabetes: it is equally important for HPs to reflect on their journey as an HP and educator. Following are some questions you might like to reflect on. It sometimes helps if you think about a person with diabetes you educated recently and felt you did not do the job as well as you would like to.

- What are your goals?
- Think about what 'do goals' influence your higher 'be goals'.
- What behaviours could be serving those goals?
- How could you learn what people with diabetes' do and be goals are?
- How could you incorporate SMARTER goals into your practice?

References

Ali S, Stone MA, Peters JL, Davies MJ, Khunti K. (2006) The prevalence of co-morbid depression in adults with Type 2 diabetes: A systematic review and meta-analysis. *Diabetic Medicine* 23(11): 1165–1173.

Anderson RM, Funnell MM. (2000) *The Art of Empowerment: Stories and Strategies for Diabetes Educators*. Alexandria, VA, American Diabetes Association.

Banks S, Dinges DF. (2007) Behavioral and physiological consequences of sleep restriction. *Journal of Clinical Sleep Medicine* 3(5):519–528.

Baran AS, Richert AC. (2003) Obstructive sleep apnoea and depression. *CNS Spectrums* 8(2):128–134.

Boulos MNK. (2005) British internet-derived patient information on diabetes mellitus: Is it readable? *Diabetes Technology & Therapeutics* 7(3):528–535.

Carver CS, Scheier MF. (2001) *On the Self-Regulation of Behavior*. Cambridge, Cambridge University Press.

Cousin N. (1979) *Anatomy of an Illness as Told by a Patient*. New York, W.W. Norton & Company.

Finnish Geriatric Intervention Study to Prevent Cognitive Impairment and Disability (FINGER) (2010) http://clinicaltrials.gov/ct2/show/NCT01041989

Friedman HS, Tucker JS, Tomlinson-Keasey C, Schwartz JE, Wingard DL, Criqui MH. (1993) Does childhood personality predict longevity? *Journal of Personality and Social Psychology*, 65:176–185.

Galliot MT, Baumeister RF. (2007) The physiology of willpower: Linking blood glucose to self-control. *Personality and Social Psychology Review* 11:303–327.

Hagger MS, Wood C, Stiff C, Chatzisarantis NL. (July 2010) Ego depletion and the strength model of self-control: A meta-analysis. *Psychological Bulletin* 136(4):495–525.

Harwood A, Harrison JE. (September 2004) How readable are orthodontic patient information leaflets? *Journal of Orthodontics* 31(3):210–219.

Kramer AF, Bherer L, Colcombe SJ. (2004) Environmental influences on cognitive and brain plasticity during aging. *Journal of Gerontology* 59A(9):940–957.

Lindberg E, Berne C, Elmasry A, Hedner J, Janson C. (2006) CPAP treatment of a population-based sample—What are the benefits and the treatment compliance? *Sleep Medicine* 7(7):553–560.

Petterson T, Dornan TL, Albert T, Lee P. (1994) Are information leaflets given to elderly people with diabetes easy to read? *Diabetic Med.* 11(1):111–113.

Van Cauter E. (2011) Sleep disturbances and insulin resistance. *Diabetic Medicine* 28:1455–1462.

Waters F, Bucks RS. (2011) Neuropsychological effects of sleep loss. *Journal of the International Neuropsychological Society* 17:571–586.

5 The Teacher: Moving from Good to Exceptional

Trisha Dunning AM

Deakin University and Barwon Health, Geelong, Victoria, Australia

> [The teacher] *If he is indeed wise he does not bid you enter the house of his wisdom, but rather leads you to the threshold of your own mind.*
> Kahlil Gibran (1883–1931)

Introduction

The purpose of Chapter 5 is to encourage diabetes educators to reflect on and challenge their notions of 'a good teacher/diabetes educator' and suggest diabetes educators owe it to people with diabetes to strive to become exceptional educators. In order to become exceptional, educators must develop extended competencies and truly understand healing and holism. But, it is difficult to define 'good' and decide when good becomes exceptional.

> *When **I** use a word*, Humpty Dumpty said in a rather scornful ton*e, it means just what I choose it to mean—neither more nor less.*
>
> *The question is*, said Alice *whether you can make words mean different things.*
>
> Lewis Carroll (1993)

So, for the time being 'good' is what the reader chooses it to mean. However, good is a value judgment that implies a linear continuum from good to bad: but people, including diabetes educators and people with diabetes, are rarely one or the other, just as HbA_{1c} is neither good nor bad: they are what they are—part of the whole picture.

Health professionals (HPs) need to consider the whole picture rather than focusing on the individual parts, because the whole reflects the sum of the parts (Bortoft 1986). One can only understand the whole by understanding the parts, that is, by taking a 'holistic' view. Holism is particularly relevant to diabetes education; for example, consider the number of parts that make up an education encounter such as the component parts of the educator and of the person with diabetes and aspects of the environment in which the encounter takes place. When the parts work together synergistically the capacity for learning is great, but if they do not, the outcomes may not suite either person, and compromise healing. Insightful educators recognise dysfunctional relationships and refer the individual to another educator.

Similarly, research that includes quantitative and qualitative aspects of the issue under study is more likely to reflect a composite or holistic view of the issues involved. For example, a randomised controlled trial of a new medicine is needed to determine effective medicine doses, dose range and dose intervals, and the safety profile. In-depth interviews using open questions will elicit participant's experience taking the medicine and the type of information people might need to take the medicine appropriately to achieve maximum benefit.

Healing

I use 'healing' deliberately: most diabetes educators know curing/treating/managing diabetes does not necessarily lead to 'good control' or optimal health, particularly when a whole person approach is not used. 'Health' comes from Anglo Saxon 'haelth' or whole; and heal from 'haelen' to restore to wholeness. Restoring to wholeness does not mean curing. It refers to mind, body and spiritual balance, accepting the situation and finding ways to move forward (transformation).

Many experts suggest the body has the capacity to heal itself, sometimes described as 'the doctor within'. The HP's role is to optimise conditions to aid the healing process. Empowering the person with diabetes is a central tenet of modern diabetes education philosophy and is linked to effective diabetes self-management (Skinner and Cradock 2000). However, if we consider Gibran's view that the teacher leads the learner to the threshold of their own mind, and the doctor within theory, 'patient empowerment' is not something educators can take sole credit for.

Educators can only create the conditions and trusting relationship within which a person with diabetes can empower themselves. Significantly, educators must be empowered themselves and competent teachers to create learning environments in which people can become whole and integrate diabetes into their lives, a process known as transformation.

Healing, in the broad context of making whole, is a social process that occurs within a therapeutic relationship (Mitchell and Cormack 1998, pp. 4–5). The healing process involves restoring the individual's sense of connectedness and control and relieving suffering, that is, to achieve balance and empowerment through holistic care (Cassell 1991). Holism recognises:

- The person's mind, body and spirit contribute to their individuality and capacity for self-empowerment and healing.
- The individual exists in a unique context: physical, social and cultural and has unique life- and diabetes-related experiences.
- The various aspects of treatment must complement each other (synergistic) to create a system where each part contributes to and enhances other parts. The educator enhances the person with diabetes' healing and self-care capacity through 'good' teaching and their way of being.
- Caring is at the heart of healing: Caring is the art that complements science. Diabetes care and education need both art and science to be holistic. Diabetes education is a complex activity. As indicated in Chapter 6, learning 'diabetes' is also a complex, lifelong activity for people with diabetes and for HPs. Caring is a highly complex phenomenon demonstrated through exceptional communication, creative care strategies, up-to-date knowledge, competence and above all the capacity to show empathy and be with the person in the moment.

Who is a teacher?

Excellent teaching is the most powerful influence on a learner's achievements (Masters 2004) and probably on teacher satisfaction and self-efficacy. 'Teach/teacher' come from the Old English 'Taecan', to show the way, point out and give instruction. Of these, 'to show the way' is the closest approximation to leading the learner to the threshold of their own mind.

Other words for teacher include Lama (Tibet), Sensi (Japan), Guru (India) and Hari Guru (Malaysia). Gurus and Sensis are known for their wisdom and authority and are revered as guides who dispel ignorance and lead people into the light. First they must achieve enlightenment themselves. The attributes of a 'good' guru are:

- Being well versed in the Vedas
- Not envying others
- Knowing yoga
- Knowing the self (self-knowledge)
- Being humble
- Practising what they preach.

In other words, a good Guru must 'have the goods' and know how to 'deliver the goods' or 'market' their message.

Attributes of a 'good' teacher

Not surprisingly, western literature indicates 'good' teachers have the same attributes as good gurus, although the language used to describe the attributes is different. A literature search of teacher attributes in 2011 yielded a great deal of information especially from school and university sources. My conversations with diabetes educator and teacher colleagues about the issue suggest diabetes educators' collective opinion is consistent with the literature as well as with the leader attributes discussed in Chapter 13. However, only a few educators mentioned leadership in the context of teaching people with diabetes.

In addition, a thematic review of Internet blogs and publications in 2011 indicates good teachers are:

- Truthful
- Passionate
- Creative
- Flexible and adaptable
- Able to integrate and build on existing information
- Connected
- Able to recognise and teach at the teachable moment
- Good role models
- Able to promote excellence
- Able to earn and give respect
- Professional.

The book, *My Favourite Teacher* (Macklin 2011) and the associated web site www.myfavouriteteacher.com.au, is a collection of the stories and recollections of 96 prominent Australians about the teachers who shaped their futures. The 'teachers' the contributors described included family members and kindergarten and primary and secondary school teachers. Contributors were men and women writers, doctors, nurses, lawyers and politicians. Sixteen key themes emerged from a structured thematic analysis of the stories that suggest the contributors remembered teachers because they:

- Loved the students and teaching and their subject
- Lit a fire rather than filled an empty vessel
- Made space for future learning (created expectation, built on existing knowledge and linked the unknown to the known)
- Were kind and respectful
- Had 'people skills'
- Used positive affirmation because it achieves more than giving negative feedback
- Were willing to go the extra mile

- Enabled students to expand their inner world
- Did something different
- Listened
- Encouraged learning partnerships and cooperation among students and between the teacher and students
- Encouraged students to consider their possibilities and options
- Understood students' cultural context
- Did not suggest what to and how to think but encouraged students *to think*
- Created an environment where learning was valued and happened
- Were able to seize the teachable moment
- Understood the power of silence: *She changed my life. And she did not say a word*

One could criticise the Internet blogs, some of the literature, informal conversations and the book as 'hearsay' rather 'true' evidence. However, careful examination shows remarkable consistency among the sources and with diabetes educator competencies promulgated by diabetes professional associations in a number of countries, for example The Australian Diabetes Educators Association (ADEA), *National Core Competencies for Credentialled Diabetes Educators* (2008). The ADEA competencies encompass the skills, knowledge, attributes, values and abilities needed to perform in five areas: person-centred diabetes care, person-centred diabetes education, organising and managing a diabetes service, professional accountability and responsibility, and leadership and patient advocacy.

Likewise, the source information for the chapter is consistent with teaching and learning theories and models (Chapter 3). Holistic teaching, teacher–learner relationships, spirituality and caring are implied in all the sources but are not prominent.

Spirituality is largely neglected in Western health care or confused with religion. Spirituality is essential to holistic care/education, empowerment, personal growth and self-efficacy. For example, young people with diabetes who regarded spirituality as an important part of their lives had lower HbA_{1c} and greater self-efficacy (Parsian and Dunning 2009). The finding is not surprising, given learning to live with diabetes is an ongoing transformational journey; transformation is at the heart of spirituality. Likewise, learning how to work with people with diabetes is part of the diabetes educator's ongoing transformational journey.

Although the attributes of 'good' diabetes educators are well documented and accepted globally, the attributes of exceptional diabetes educators are less clear. Some might regard credentialing/certification as evidence of exceptional practice; however, it is not clear that credentialed/certified diabetes educators actually perform differently from non-credentialled/certified diabetes educators, nor that core competencies reflect the competencies needed for exceptional practice.

Moving from good to exceptional

Once we accept our limits we go beyond them.

Albert Einstein (1879–1951)

The difference between good and exceptional diabetes educators may be recognising and going beyond individual limits. Exceptional educators are proficient in the core competences and have the required attributes. In addition they:

- Have a philosophy of diabetes care and education.
- Value and actively develop a therapeutic relationship with each individual they teache (people with diabetes and HPs).
- Know the self.
- Reflect in and on practice, individually or within communities of learning.
- Have the ability to be present with the individual in the moment.
- Take care of the self.

Philosophy of diabetes care and education

The following philosophy was generated from my personal upbringing, culture, learning, experience and other life influences. It evolved over time, and is likely to continue to evolve as I learn, and hopefully continue to grow. I have never discussed or shared my philosophy before; so I share it here with some trepidation.

- Diabetes education is not an isolated activity. It occurs within life and social contexts. It is a lifelong, continuous process of transformation for people with diabetes and diabetes educators.
- People with diabetes are diverse and have a range of experiences, self-knowledge and capabilities. They are entitled to individualised, holistic care and education that encompasses mind, body and spirit that maintains hope.
- Educators must know themselves, their capabilities and limitations, values, beliefs and attitudes in order to care for and teach others.
- In order to know themselves and improve practice, educators must be open-minded and reflect on each experience to achieve personal growth as part of continual professional development. They must look within and outside their profession for information and inspiration.
- Exceptional diabetes education is a creative blend of art and science. People with diabetes are entitled to best practice evidence-based care delivered using a range of creative strategies.

- Educators have an obligation to be effective, caring, holistic and professional, by practising within the limits of their knowledge and competence, role and scope of practice, legislation and regulatory frameworks, and codes of conduct and ethics and being aware of professional boundaries within consultations.
- Educators have an obligation to demonstrate leadership in teaching and practice by acting as role models, contributing to research, the profession and the community and the interdisciplinary team.
- Focusing on the positive and giving positive feedback are key empowering strategies.
- Sustaining hope is important to an individual's self-care, self-concept and self-efficacy. Sustaining hope does not mean hope for a cure for diabetes.
- Educators must respect people's learning styles, beliefs, attitudes, goals and explanatory models and do their best to accommodate them, be non-judgmental, use congruent teaching, optimal communication, openness and acceptance.
- Teaching and learning is an interrelated process where mutual learning occurs.
- Learning and self-growth can only occur within a trusting therapeutic relationship. In such a relationship people learn from each other.
- Effective communication is essential to establishing and maintaining therapeutic relationships. Effective communication includes verbal, written, body language, gestures, paralingual speech, active listening and silence.
- People's stories are valuable. They provide essential information that enables educators to understand people's life experiences, goals, attitudes and beliefs and the language they use. Stories help educators develop strategies to enhance people with diabetes' self-concept and capabilities.
- Educators must create an environment where the individual feels safe to share their story recognising that they might disclose information that should remain confidential unless the individual agrees it can be disclosed (excluding mandatory reportable information).
- Educators can only create such an environment if they are present in the moment. In order to be present in the moment, educators must be connected and engaged on several levels: with the self, with the individual or group, the profession, the organisation and team the educator works in, and society/community.
- Educators must be skilled salespeople to market the product 'diabetes', a product most people would prefer not buy. Such marketing must be honest and accurate and disclose benefits, risks and costs. Diabetes educators can learn marketing skills from business models.

- It is important to evaluate outcomes and personal performance using appropriate valid tools/methods. Reflection in and on practice is part of personal evaluation.
- Exceptional diabetes educators, like exceptional leaders, are politically aware and advocate for and with people with diabetes.
- To sustain such a philosophy, diabetes educators must be committed, passionate and self-caring, that is, they have a responsibility to nurture the self.

Factors that influence philosophy

Each diabetes educator will have their own unique philosophy, even if it is not clearly articulated or documented. Many diabetes educators will recognise some elements in my philosophy they can relate to because we share similar training and clinical experiences, no matter where we worked or trained.

Elements of my philosophy originated within my family and at school. My father taught me to love books, my mother to care and contribute to the community. Two general practitioners (GPs), Drs Cookson and Holmes, who worked in the country town where I grew up, went to school, and trained as a nurse, lived and role modelled a philosophy I embraced. There were no house officers, consultant specialists or medical students in the town. Thus, the GPs had a very close working relationship with the nurses and relied on their expertise. GPs and nurses were closely connected to and were part of community in which they delivered care. There were five others in my training group. Drs Cookson and Holmes loved teaching.

About 3 months after I commenced my training, Dr Cookson said:

I see you have a day off tomorrow. I will pick you up at nine. Be on time.

I was about to protest when he said:

I am doing my home visits. I only need about an hour of your time. If you don't know where these patients come from, their home situations, their relationships and pets, how will you plan their discharge and know they will be able to manage when they go home? How will you understand their stories?

Shortly after that he 'invited' me to a post-mortem: '*You need to know how bodies go together to understand people's diseases so you can provide good nursing care like preventing pressure sores*'.

Both doctors insisted trainee nurses accompanied them on ward rounds—usually the prerogative of the 'Sister'. They discussed people's diseases, social situations, mental health and medical and nursing care. We learned in 'real time' and could apply the information immediately, which reinforced learning. They were masters at teaching at the teachable moment.

There was a standard curriculum and competencies that trainee nurses had to complete, but Drs Cookson and Holmes believed we learned more in the 'teachable moment' than 'slavishly following the book'. We did complete all that was required and it did not seem to matter that the learning did not proceed in the sequence set out in the curriculum. We learned to assess, observe, listen, use all five senses, ask questions and reflect so we could make connections and recognise patterns that enable us to apply the knowledge in other situations.

The doctors insisted good medicine and good nursing were a blend of art and science and practitioner behaviours. They set 'homework' after teaching rounds from the prescribed textbooks and other relevant research they found, and, very exiting for me (but not all my fellow trainees), novels and poetry. Later, they asked us about the characters in the books: what motivated them, what shaped their characters and what could be applied to nursing care.

Three weeks before the final exams, the Drs asked Matron to arrange a meeting with the five finalists, where they announced:

> The five of you sitting finals will be working morning shifts for the next three weeks. At six o'clock you will come to my house or Charlie's [Dr Holmes]. Our wives will make dinner and we will revise, debate, question and clarify so you are all as well prepared for the finals as you can possibly be.

These two doctors embodied Gray's observation that:

> The physician, if he is properly educated to his profession must be familiar with many parts of his nature, philosophy, with natural history, botany, chemistry as well as with those branches of learning which more immediately connect themselves with the science of life and the knowledge of disease.
>
> Gray (Undated)

The same could be said of any HP, especially exceptional HPs.

Later, many colleagues were role models for diabetes education, clinical care and research. People with diabetes and their relatives taught and continue to teach me about life with diabetes, which enriches my philosophy.

Therapeutic relationship

A respectful therapeutic relationship is essential to achieving optimal outcomes (Heine 1981; Hamburg and Inoff 1982; Bennett-Levy 2006). Significantly, the strength of the therapeutic relationship is a strong predictor of outcomes. Effective communication is the key to developing therapeutic relationships.

Bordin's (1979) definition of therapeutic relationship or alliance is still used. Bordin defined three interrelated components:

- HP and individual agreement about treatment goals
- HP and individual agreement about how to achieve the goals
- A personal bond between the HP and the individual

The way an educator establishes a relationship with an individual is critical to the outcome of the relationship. The educator must be willing to share power and earn the individual's trust before good communication and learning can take place. Diabetes educators must actively develop skills that will enable them to develop relationships. These skills include:

- Caring, which is an interpersonal process that generates a caring moment that enhances the likelihood of positive outcomes for both people in the relationship
- Accepting without judgment or blame
- Demonstrating respect
- Showing empathy, which requires active listening and understanding
- Listening, attending and actively involving the individual in the conversation
- Being truly present in the consultation by paying close attention (attending)
- Asking open questions to encourage dialogue
- Clarifying responses and reflecting people's responses
- Using silence
- Being connected
- Providing support
- Effectively and appropriately using language including body language and respecting personal space and verbal, spatial and behavioural boundaries
- Promoting equality
- Being professional (Mitchell and Cormack 1998; Dziopa and Ahern 2009).

Establishing relationships can be challenging, even when the educator is experienced and skilled, especially within the time constraints and other barriers:

- Characteristics of the individuals involved
- Competing priorities of both individuals
- Waiting times
- Consultation environment, e.g. privacy can be compromised in shared hospital rooms
- Time pressures
- Interruptions during consultations

- Organisational imperatives and expectations
- Nature of the information disclosed and shared.

Likewise, there are many missed opportunities to establish relationship, for example the exchange in Chapter 6 under the subheading 'voices' is an opportunity to 'seize the day'. Currently, many HPs caring for people with diabetes focus on diabetes, rather than the person with diabetes. The biomedical focus could be partly due to current guidelines and care algorithms that outline care pathways, medicines and medical care, but rarely include the art of care, and often collect closed information by 'ticking boxes' (Chapter 13).

Listening

Listening is essential to developing therapeutic relationships and is a particular skill. People with diabetes spend most of the time in medical and education encounters listening. Ideally, the situation should be reversed because people only remember a fraction of what they are told.

A great deal of effort and concentration is needed to actively listen. Active listening involves the listener:

- Receiving aural input
- Interpreting the message in light of their background, existing knowledge and experience
- Understanding the language the speaker uses.

Information is initially processed as it is being received. People are still processing the information they just heard, when the next piece arrives. In addition, listeners (educators and people with diabetes) have to adapt to the speaker's language and delivery mode (Chapter 6). People with low literacy levels, those who speak different languages and people with hearing deficits find listening challenging and often stop listening.

Different sorts of information require different listening skills; for example 'How are you?' is less demanding on the listener then a long speech that contains multiple pieces of information that might be new or not relevant to the listener, or out of context.

Becoming an exceptional diabetes educator is part of the educator's transformational journey. Transformation occurs through self-knowledge and reflection.

Know yourself

An HP's duty of care includes knowing the limits of their knowledge and competence. Self-knowledge, like education, is a journey towards ways of seeing and being in the world.

Understanding the self requires self-honesty, reflection and willingness to change. Teaching, like other human activities, emerges from within the educator. If a teacher is willing to critically review their performance, they have a chance of increasing self-knowledge.

Knowing myself is as crucial to good teaching as knowing my students and my subject. In fact, knowing students depends on self-knowledge. If I do not know my students I cannot teach well.

Palmer (1998, p. 2)

Many educators engage in 'self-talk' after a teaching encounter, usually when things do not go well. That is not genuine self-reflection and rarely improves practice, essentially because knowledge of self does not change, therefore, nothing else changes. When things do not work, the educator needs to change what they are doing. Deep self-questioning can be confronting and can be undertaken alone. Alternatively, objective peer-review that focuses on the behaviour not the person, constructive patient evaluation and mentoring relationships can aid self-knowledge.

Some personal attributes educators could consider are:

Emotional intelligence: A set of essential individual human capacities that shape the individual's ability to manage their emotions and develop positive relationships (Goleman 1995).

Social intelligence: Human brains are hard-wired to connect with other people. That is, humans are innately social beings. Relationships shape people's experiences and biology: nourishing relationships have a beneficial effect on health; toxic or demoralising relationships affect physical, mental and spiritual health (Goleman 2007, p. 5).

Multiple intelligence: The Theory of Multiple Intelligences (Gardner 1983) is widely used but is sometimes criticised as being rhetoric rather than evidence. Gardner believed people have different capacities for performing different activities and described eight categories of intelligence:

- Linguistic—using and understanding language
- Logical mathematical—mathematical ability and ability to see patterns and be analytical and scientific
- Musical—appreciation of musical, hearing tones and rhythms
- Bodily—kinaesthetic-body awareness, know how bodies work
- Spatial—knowledge of distance and space and spatial relationships
- Interpersonal—understanding other people including non-verbal language and own capabilities and limitations
- Naturalist—recognise and categorise things
- Existential or spiritual—self-knowledge and personal growth.

The Theory of Multiple Intelligences has been used to describe learning styles to help teachers plan teaching strategies to match the learning style (see Chapters 3 and 13). People may have one preferred 'intelligence style', but they can develop several styles to suit different learning situations: educators who develop a spectrum of 'intelligences' may be more competent at engaging with and forming relationships with people with diabetes, than educators who do not.

Wounded healer

Some educators may not be familiar with 'wounded healer' theories. The concept is relevant to all educators but may be particularly applicable to diabetes educators who have diabetes. Basically, when an individual experiences a 'wound', which might be trauma, diagnosis of a disease such as diabetes, a mental disorder or loss, they pass through stages of healing/recovery: wounded, walking wounded and wounded healer and when they are healed they transcend the wound (Conti-O'Hare 2002).

Wounded healers develop significant self-knowledge and can use their experience constructively to help other people. People who have not commenced the healing process and the walking wounded may suffer emotional distress when they encounter other people with the same condition, or develop enmeshed and/or non-productive relationships that result in miscarried helping (Anderson and Coyne 1991).

In the end, only the wounded physician heals and even he, in the last analysis, cannot heal beyond the extent to which he has healed himself (van der Post 1975).

Reflection

Reflection is essential to continued professional development and exceptional diabetes education. Schon (1983) presented a model for reflective practice that is still relevant. He observed that when effective practitioners were faced with a problem, they instinctively drew on previous experience, recognised patterns and considered various solutions, which he called reflection-in-action (reflection during the event). He suggested that learning could be enhanced by reflection-on-action (reflection after the event). Further, Schon believed the ability to reflect both in and on action distinguishes 'effective from less effective practitioners'.

Reflection-on-action can occur individually or in groups such as case studies and when evaluating critical incidents. Group reflection enables educators to examine the link between abstract knowledge, information learned but not used in practice and actual practice. Schon's work highlights the importance of practical experience to the learning process.

Practical experience also teaches us to learn from mistakes and that simple strategies are often the most effective, as the Sorcerer's apprentice found out when he tried out his magic skills on the brooms when the sorcerer was away. The brooms became uncontrollable, very disobedient and created havoc in the house: *Desist broom* the apprentice repeatedly cried to no avail. The sorcerer returned, stared at the mess and said *stop!* And the broom did.

Reflection in and on practice can help diabetes educators:

- Record and explore experiences and learn from them.
- Enhance their problem-solving skills.
- Explore personal beliefs, attitudes and explanatory models.
- Evaluate performance.
- Acquire self-knowledge and enhance professional practice.
- Enhance continuing professional development activities (Moon 1999). In fact, reflection will be mandatory when the revised ADEA continuing professional development process is implemented later in 2012.

Educators could help people with diabetes use reflection in and on their diabetes self-care behaviours and outcomes during consultations, since reflection is essentially a problem-solving technique. Likewise, reflection could be a useful strategy to actively involve people in the consultation.

Being present in the moment

Effective education is more likely when the educator is fully engaged, actively listening and connected (present). The phenomenon is sometimes referred to as authentic presence (Newman 2008). Being present is also a form of accompaniment or witnessing that can help people come to terms with their diagnosis, even when they do not understand the disease or its treatment (Weingarten 2004). Significantly, being fully present is essential to establishing effective relationships.

The educator can demonstrate authentic presence by being attentive, open and focused on the individual. People are more likely to share their stories and explanatory models and disclose key information if the educator is fully present, because presence nurtures hope.

Self-care

Diabetes education is emotionally and physically demanding. Exceptional practice is only possible if the educator manages stress, lives a healthy lifestyle, that is, lives what they preach and heal their own wounds.

Summary

'Good' worked very hard in this chapter and

That's a great deal to make one word mean said Alice in a thoughtful tone. *When I make a word do a lot of work like that said* Humpty Dumpty *I always pay it extra.*

Lewis Carroll (1993)

People with diabetes are likely to benefit when diabetes educators move from being good to being exceptional teachers. Learning to be an exceptional educator is a transformational journey. The more educators learn about themselves and the more they reflect on and develop their knowledge and skills, the more effective they will be.

Reflective questions

Reflection is essential to learning. It is a key part of the person with diabetes' journey and it is equally important for HPs to reflect on their journey as carers and educators. The following statements or questions may help you reflect. It sometimes helps if you think about a recent encounter with a person with diabetes where you felt the encounter did not go as well as you would like.

- Do you have a personal diabetes care and educational philosophy?
- Is it written down anywhere?
- What factors shaped your philosophy?
- Are you a 'wounded healer'? If so, did the experience help you grow as a diabetes educator?
- How could you apply the Theory of Multiple Intelligences to diabetes education?

References

Anderson B, Coyne J. (1991) Miscarried helping in families of children and adolescents with chronic diseases. In Johns J, Johnson B (eds.), *Advances in Child Health Psychology*. Gainesville, FL, University of Florida.

Australian Diabetes Educators Association (ADEA). (2008) *National Core Competencies fro Credentialled Diabetes Educators*. Canberra, Australian Capital Territory, Australia, ADEA.

Bennett-Levy J. (2006) Self and self-reflection in the therapeutic relationship: A conceptual map and practical strategies for the training, supervision and self-preservation of interpersonal skills. In Chapter 12, Gilbert P, Leahy R (eds.), *The Therapeutic Relationship in the Cognitive-Behavioural Psychotherapies*. London, Routledge.

Bordin E. (1979) The generalisability of the psychoanalytic concept of the working alliance in psychotherapy. *Research and Practice* 16:252–260.

Bortoft H. (1986) *Goethe's Scientific Consciousness*. Kent, England, Institute for Cultural Research (Monograph Series 22).

Carroll L. (1993, first published 1871) *Through the Looking Glass—What Alice Found There*. London, Harpur Collins.

Cassell E. (1991) *The Nature of Suffering and the Goals of Medicine*. Oxford, Oxford University Press.

Conti-O'Hare M. (2002) *The Nurse as Wounded Healer*. Boston, MA, Jones and Bartlett Publishers.

Dziopa F, Ahern K. (2009) What makes a quality therapeutic relationship in psychiatric/mental health nursing: A review of the research literature. *The Internet Journal of Advanced Nursing Practice* 10(1):1–19.

Gardner H. (1983) Howard Gardner's theory of multiple intelligences summarised by Sandra Dodd. http://sandradodd.com/intelligences (accessed March 2010).

Gibran K. (2008) *Kahlil Gibran's the Prophet and the Art of Peace*. The New Illustrated Edition. London, Duncan Baird Publishers p. 99.

Goleman D. (1995) *Emotional Intelligence*. New York, Bantam Books.

Goleman D. (2007) *Social Intelligence*. London, Arrow Books, pp. 4–5.

Gray F. (date unknown) *North American Review*. Vol. xxii, New Series. Boston, MA.

Hamburg B, Inoff G. (1982) Relationship between behavioural factors and diabetic control in children and adolescents: A camp study. *Psychosomatic Medicine* 44:321–339.

Heine A. (1981) Helping hypertensive clients help themselves: The nurse's role. *Patient Education and Counselling* 3(July–September):108–112.

Macklin R. (2011) *My Favourite Teacher*. Sydney, New South Wales, Australia, University of New South Wales Press.

Masters G. (2004) What makes a good teacher? *Education Review* 7(3): 452–466.

Mitchell A, Cormack M. (1998) *The Therapeutic Relationship in Complementary Health Care*. London, Churchill Livingstone.

Moon J. (1999) *Reflections in Learning and Professional Development: Theory and Practice*. Herndon, VA, Stylus Publishing.

Newman M. (2008) *Transforming Presence*. Philadelphia, PA, E.A. Davis, p. 51.

Palmer P. (1998) *The Courage to Teach: Exploring the Inner Landscape of a Teacher's life*. San Francisco, CA, Jossey Bass.

Parsian N, Dunning T. (2009) Spirituality—An important aspect of care in young adults with diabetes. *The Australian Diabetes Educator* 12(1):10–11 and 16.

van der Post L. (1975) *Jung and the Story of our Time*. New York, Random House.

Schon D. (1983) Educating the reflective practitioner. Site updated on November 2000. http://edu.queensu.ca/~russellt/howteach/schon87.htm (accessed July 2011).

Skinner T, Cradock S. (2000) Empowerment: What about the evidence. *Practical Diabetes International* 17(3):91–99.

Weingarten K. (2004) Commentary: What is at the centre, what the edges of care? *Family, Systems, Medicine* 22:151–157.

6 People Do Not Always Speak the Same Language Even When They Speak the Same Language

Trisha Dunning AM

Deakin University and Barwon Health, Geelong, Victoria, Australia

> *Telling stories about illness is to give voice to the body ... the body
> sets in motion the need for new stories when disease disrupts old stories.*
>
> Frank (1995)

Introduction

Many of my colleagues will be pleased to know Chapter 6 does not address the grammar and structure of language: that is, it is not concerned with *The cold blooded murder of the English tongue* (Professor Henry Higgins, *My Fair Lady*), although I have done my best to preserve the English tongue— you will not find any 'weasel words' (Watson 2004), tense disagreement, dangling participles, split infinitives or 'undefined this', in my chapters. Likewise, the chapter does not concern linguistics. It discusses the power and drama of language, what language is, how it shapes people's thoughts and behaviours, and the social context in which language is used.

What is language?

It should be easy to provide a precise definition of 'language', but definitions differ depending on whom one asks. For example, The *Shorter Oxford Dictionary* provides several meanings for 'language' including:

> *The whole body of words and methods of combining them used by a nation, people or race. A method of expression other than by words.... Ability to speak a foreign tongue ... style of composition.*

Diabetes Education: Art, Science and Evidence, First Edition. Edited by Trisha Dunning AM.
© 2013 John Wiley & Sons, Ltd. Published 2013 by John Wiley & Sons, Ltd.

Writers, philosophers and linguists use other 'definitions', for example:

- *Speech is a complex activity encompassing the means of persuasion, the language and the proper arrangement of the various parts of the speech.* (Aristotle translated by Roberts 1954).
- *Language is the dress of thought.* (Samuel Johnson's 1709–1784 translation of Quintillian's witticism).
- *Language is a collection and unconscious art.* (Charles Darwin 1871)
- *The shape of thought.* (Whorf 1956).
- *To write jargon is like perpetually shuffling around in the fog and cotton wool of abstract terms.* (Sir Arthur Quiller-Couch 1916).

The last comment is particularly pertinent to diabetes education. If we do not use clear, unambiguous language, written and spoken, tailored to the particular individual or group, they will 'shuffle around in the fog' and the educator may not even be aware the fog exists. Creating fog is particularly easy when the educator and the person with diabetes do not speak the same language or have different literacy and numeracy skills, goals and experiences of diabetes (see Chapter 13). Recognising and clearing the fog relies on excellent communication skills to arrive at a shared understanding/meaning.

A composite definition of language might be:

The process humans use to communicate thoughts, feelings and ideas using voice, sounds, gestures and written or pictorial symbols. The system includes rules for combining components such as words, gestures (coverbal behaviours), paralingual sounds (phonetics), and body language to arrive at a shared understanding or common meaning.

Different parts of the brain are involved in different aspects of language. Damage in any of these areas could affect other areas and communication:

- Wernicke's area — Comprehension
- Upper temporal lobe — Auditory reception
- Broca's area in the frontal lobe — Encoding speech
- Exner's area in the frontal lobe — Motor control of writing
- Part of the parietal lobe — Manual signing
- Occipital lobe — Visual input (Crystal 2006, pp. 171–179)

In addition, the mid-superior temporal sulcus, rostral prefrontal cortex and the frontal and temporal cortex are involved with social cognition. These regions are important for a variety of communication behaviours such as interpreting facial expressions, gestures, theory of mind and predicting the behaviour of other people (Johnson 2011).

Components of language

The main components of language are speech, gestures, paralingual sounds, and body language.

Paralingual sounds

Paralingual sounds (sometimes called phonetics) are vocal noises superimposed on speech. They have some, but not all, of the properties of language, for example laughing and crying while speaking (Crystal 2006, p. 14). Paralingual sounds add 'emotional colour' to speech to make it more interesting. Paralingual sounds serve a similar purpose to gestures and body language. One can almost hear the paralingual sounds in some writing, particularly when it is spoken, for example many Dr Seuss books.

Gestures

Humans use many gestures to communicate and emphasise spoken language; although gestures are a form of sign language, few have a formal structure and range. Auslan, a sign language, does have a defined structure and complexity. Different gestures and symbols have different meanings in different cultures and languages.

Speakers use several types of gestures:

- Emblems/symbolic gestures, many of which are universally understood such as 'thumbs up'.
- Batons/beats, simple repetitive rhythmic hand movements that coordinate with the tempo of the sentence.
- Gesticulations, which often accompany spontaneous speech. Gesticulations vary and are usually non-repetitive and might be related to the content of the message (Krauss and Chiu 1997).

Diabetes educators could use relevant gestures to support and emphasise diabetes education messages, but overuse can be distracting and defeat the purpose.

Words

Words are a key aspect of language in addition to gestures and paralingual sounds, and can be spoken or written. Words are just nouns, pronouns, verbs, adjectives or adverbs until the writer, speaker and listener give them meaning, but the meaning each person attaches to the word, might be, and often is, different. In addition, meaning is influenced by whether and how the word is spoken or written and environmental and other factors such as body language, which is discussed later in the chapter.

Spoken

The speaker's voice (diction, tone, pitch, range), speaking speed, where the speaker places the emphasis, punctuation, where and how words fit in the speech, paralingual sounds, gestures, the personal meaning individuals attach to the word(s), their culture, education and literacy level, feelings at the time, health status and culture affect the way language is interpreted.

Listener characteristics: all of the speaker characteristics as well as hearing acuity, interest in the topic, concentration span, listening skills and learning style.

Environment: noise, privacy and other distractions.

Written

Written words can be inert, ambiguous or very clear, depending on how the sentences are constructed and the 'signposts' the writer uses to help the reader find meaning in the text. Passive language and weasel words are more likely to be ambiguous than active, clear writing. Examples of passive language abound in many government documents, just watch any episode of *Yes Minister* or listen to parliamentarians being interviewed on the news. Weasel words can be useful if the intention is to create fog and confuse, or reduce tension and slow the pace in fiction writing, but they usually do not belong in diabetes education information.

'Signpost' in the context of writing refers to punctuation, headings, subheadings, design and layout, which help the reader navigate the text. Grammar and words can have a profound effect on how people see the world (Boroditsky 2003) and by extension, their diabetes. Significantly, people who speak different languages think differently.

Thus, words come alive in the minds of the individual, or they are discarded if the word is not understood or the individual is not interested in the topic. Words can be the starting point in a conversation, or a conversation stopper. They can help people assemble information they already know, or trigger new learning, which has important implications for both spoken and written diabetes education information.

Learning a language

Learning any language is not easy, except for children! Consider the word 'diabetes'. Most diabetes educators know it is derived from the Greek word for 'siphon'. However, most people diagnosed with diabetes have to learn a lot of words related to diabetes, such that it could be considered a 'language or dialect' in its own right. Diabetes is a very complex language, and like all languages, it constantly evolves as new words are added and old ones are discarded.

Diabetes educators have to learn 'diabetes' initially and then keep up-to-date with the evolving language. But do diabetes educators and people with diabetes speak the same diabetes language/dialect?

Can you understand the following Old English verse from Beowulf?

Alegdon tha middes maerne theoden
Haeleth hiofende hlaford leofne
Ongunnon tha on beorge bael-fyra maest
Wigend weccan wudu-rec astah
Sweart ofer swiothhole swogende leg
Wope bewunden

Perhaps modern English is easier:

The sorrowing soldiers then laid the glorious prince, their dear lord, in the middle. Then on the hill the war-men began to light the greatest of funeral fires. The wood-smoke rose black above the flames, the noisy fire, mixed with sorrowful cries.

Chickman and Howett (2006)

Did you try to understand the Old English or give up because it is not relevant to you and you are not interested in it anyway? Did you 'cheat' and read the modern English version? If you could read it, it tells you quite a lot about how the soldiers regarded their dead Prince and their funeral rites. Likewise, written diabetes information generally contains a lot of information about diabetes, but unless the individual can read and understand it easily, is interested in it and it is relevant to their needs at the time, they are likely to ignore it.

A great deal of 'diabetes' reflects the biomedical language of health professionals (HPs) rather than the psychosocially oriented language people with diabetes use. When relating to people with diabetes, HPs often only hear the former. When that happens, there is a mismatch between what the individual wants to know or discuss and what HPs want to know and discuss (Scheeres et al. 2008).

The power of language

Language is so powerful that the major cause of health-related critical incidents and complaints about HPs are the result of ineffective communication on the part of HPs. Not recognising the importance of language and culture can result in health-related problems, inhibit a person's ability to provide informed consent and understand and accept a diagnosis and treatment, dissatisfaction with care, and preventable morbidity and mortality (Flores et al. 2002).

Language in the broadest context influences the way people:

- Perceive and remember events
- Make decisions about causality
- Understand written and spoken materials and numbers
- Perceive and experience emotion
- Choose to take risks
- Think about other people (Boroditsky 2003).

When people learn a new language they also learn new ways of thinking. Thus, the language(s) people speak has a profound effect on the way they think, view the world and live their lives, and can affect the people around them.

The book *The Uncommon Reader* (Bennett 2007) is a fictitious account of the profound effect a chance encounter with a mobile library had on Queen Elizabeth II. The Queen became obsessed with books. The story traces the consequences of her obsession on her family, her advisers, who, among other things, had to warn the public: 'Her Majesty will probably ask you what you are reading'. The obsession even threatens her position as Queen. Over 20 books are mentioned in the novella.

The title is a play on the word 'common', which has several meanings in English: vulgar, ordinary and anybody who is not royal or of noble birth. But how does Queen Elizabeth's reading habits relate to diabetes? Consider the Diabetes Australia (DA) (2011) *Position Statement: A New Language for Diabetes*. The Statement highlights the effect language and words can have on an individual's health, self-identity and self-efficacy, and suggests some ways people with diabetes could interpret words like 'disease', 'failed', 'blood tests' and 'compliance' and recommends some alternatives.

Readers will note I was deliberately non-compliant with the Position Statement recommendations in Chapter 11: I choose to use the words 'compliant' and 'non-complaint' with respect to medicine use. These words embody far more complex behaviours/issues than is apparent on first reading the words. Compliance and non-compliance were more appropriate in Chapter 11 than many of the current euphemisms. HPs are not immune to non-compliance!

Hitler's Private Library: The Books That Shaped His Life (Ryback 2009) is an account of the books that shaped Hitler's thoughts and deeds—fascinating, considering Hitler is renowned for burning books. Hitler's book choices are interesting, and his handwritten notes, comments in the margins and underlined passages of text tell the reader a lot about how the words affected him and shaped the dictator he became. A lot of the text Hitler highlighted, and his margin notes, are evident in his speeches.

Hitler is quoted as saying '… I take what I want from books' (Ryback 2009, p. xi). Hitler ranked the *Collected Works of Shakespeare, Don Quixote,* and *Uncle Tom's Cabin* among the greatest works of world literature. In addition, he owned many works by German writers and other world philosophers including von Goethe.

Anybody reading my writing can see books have a powerful influence on my thinking and philosophy, including my philosophy of diabetes education (Chapter 3). I am a voracious reader, and love good writing. I get enormous pleasure from creative and academic writing. Like Hitler, I write notes in book margins and underline or highlight text, I too 'take what I want from books', but there the comparison ends!

People with diabetes also 'take what they want' from written and spoken information diabetes educators provide, they highlight and use what is interesting and relevant to them and discard the rest. Thus, the individual with diabetes has control over whether and how they use information. However, not all language is verbal or written: body language plays a major role in communication.

Body language

Body language is a sophisticated language that emerged before spoken language (Eggert 2010). Complicated messages can be communicated via body language, just think of mimes and charades. Likewise, babies have different cries to signify hunger or discomfort. Some body language is universal, but most people develop their own body language style, which is influenced by their culture, upbringing, role models, manners and etiquette, experience and social environment. Thus, the more time a diabetes educator spends with an individual, the better they will understand them.

Body language acts as a catalyst between the words people say and the full meaning they wish to convey. Thus, body language helps give colour, drama and meaning to spoken language. Some experts believe humans are programmed to use and understand basic body language (Ekman 1982), which helps people respond to the situation, for example when it is another person's turn to speak, or when the individual does not understand what was said. However, it is essential to listen, check assumptions and consider cultural differences, rather than jumping to conclusions or speaking at cross-purposes.

Body language refers to the unconscious movements people make while thinking, speaking and listening. Often the individual is unaware of their body language; at other times they use it deliberately. Mehrabian (1971) said there are three main components of face-to-face communication and indicated the percent contribution of each component to the communication:

1. What is said, 7%
2. How it is said, 38%

3. Facial expressions of both communicators, 55%. Other researchers dispute these percentages; nonetheless, there is an important message for diabetes educators about the relative impact of the various speech components.

Sometimes the body language does not match what the individual says (incongruence). To achieve clear communication, spoken and body language must be congruent. Diabetes educators automatically 'scan' colleagues and people with diabetes and make decisions about them based on facial expressions, body language and demeanour or other HPs' notes or comments, which influences clinical and education encounters.

Diabetes educators also need to appreciate that people with diabetes are often under stress and vulnerable during education and clinical assessments, for example when they is diagnosed (Chapter 2) and during hospital admissions. People are also vulnerable to conflicting and/or misleading information. Diabetes educators may not be able to control all aspects of the communication, for example constant interruptions when 'at the bedside'.

Many factors influence body language: diabetes educators need to be very careful not to misinterpret other people's body language and be sure their own spoken and body language is congruent to avoid miscommunication. It is important to watch for clusters of body movements rather than basing an assumption on one movement. Observing clusters of body language and congruence with speech can help educators understand what other people actually mean.

Michael Solomon, Chairman of the Graduate School of Business NYU suggested people make 11 decisions about a person in the first 7 s of contact. Subsequent researchers suggest such decisions are made in the first one tenth of a second and include decisions about economic level, education level, honesty, sexual orientation, values, ethnicity and social standing. In addition, a great deal of the time in the subsequent conversation is spent trying to find evidence to support the first impression (Willis and Todorov 2006).

Some recent Australian 'social research' involved well-known television reporters portraying different characters, including a well-dressed frail older lady, a homeless person and a well-dressed businessman. The public responded most favourably to the well-dressed businessman than the other characters. The research is not conclusive but suggests we need to heed the old adages 'there is more to people than meets the eye' and 'don't jump to conclusions'.

The message is clear for diabetes educators: the first impression the person with diabetes/carers forms of the educator can influence the rest of the education encounter. First impressions can change as people spend more time together; but, given the time constraints in many diabetes services, the educator may not get a second chance. Therefore, the first impression you make must count. Some tips for maximising the positive aspects of the first impression are shown in Box 6.1.

> **Box 6.1   Tips that can help diabetes educators make a favourable first impression on people with diabetes, their carers and colleagues**
>
> - Dress appropriately in clothes you like and feel comfortable but mindful that being seen to be part of the group is important (see Chapter 13). People communicate through dress in many ways. Consider Mark Twain's comments: 'Clothes make the man' and 'Naked people have little or no influence on society' and Herbert Vreeland's observation that 'Clothes don't make the man, but clothes have got many a man a job'
> - Be mindful of your body language. Make sure it is culturally relevant and congruent. Since body language is mostly unconscious. The diabetes educator will need to be very aware of their first reactions to other people
> - Start the conversation in a positive, truthful manner
> - Maintain social eye contact to convey interest, honesty and to indicate you are listening
> - Smile to show personal warmth
> - Consider whether a handshake is appropriate. My father-in-law maintained you can 'Tell the character of a man by the strength of his handshake'. I later learned that it is not true in many cultures where a hand touch or limp handshake is appropriate and a firm handshake is bad manners. Nodding or bowing might be more appropriate in some cultures
> - Lean forward slightly when you speak to indicate friendship but be mindful of the other person's personal space
> - Mirror the other person's body language to build trust and rapport. The closer the mirroring, the closer the rapport (Lakin 2003)
> - Always check your first impressions, look for 'evidence' in the information the individual shares, ask relevant questions and listen carefully to the answers

Culture

Language is shaped by and reflects culture. According to the Talmud, there are four languages worth using: Greek for song, Latin for war, Syriac for lamentation and Hebrew for ordinary speech. Likewise, the Holy Roman Emperor, Charles V King of Spain and Archduke of Austria, who spoke several languages, said he spoke 'Spanish to God, Italian to women, French to men and German to his horse' (Deutscher 2010, p. 1). These two examples show how people automatically adapt their language to the person or context.

They are salutary lessons for diabetes educators, who educate and care for people with diabetes from diverse backgrounds, experiences and cultures.

There are a number of peculiarities among languages that could affect how people with diabetes learn. For example, some languages do not have a future tense, which makes the concept of 'developing diabetes in the future' and 'long-term goals' difficult for them to understand. Some languages use the same word for hand and fingers, which can lead to confusion about where to prick the 'finger' when performing a blood glucose test.

The Kuuk Thaayorre, a small Australian Aboriginal community in Cape York in Northern Australia, relate spatially to the cardinal directions, north, south, east and west, whereas English speakers tend to say right, left, backwards and forwards. Needless to say, the Kuuk Thaayorre have a better sense of direction than most English speakers, but the same might not be true of urban-dwelling Aboriginals, who have less need to orient according to the cardinal points. Knowing such information is important to selecting appropriate words for specific contexts.

Similarly, English speakers refer to time in terms of length, e.g. 'a long walk'; Spanish and Greek speakers talk about time in amounts, e.g. 'big' and 'little' rather than 'short' and 'long'. Mandarin speakers describe time vertically, e.g. the next month is the 'down month' and the preceding month was the 'up month' (Boroditsky 2003; Deutscher 2010). It is easy to see how people can become confused when they do not speak the same language or come from different cultures. Such facts highlight the wisdom of Talmud and the Holy Roman Emperor who adapted their language to suit the person they were communicating with.

Globalisation, technology, wars and natural disasters have a significant effect on migration, planned and refugees, such that language and word usage are evolving rapidly (Erard 2008). Not being able to communicate in the same language as the person with diabetes is a challenge for many diabetes educators. Culture is a barrier to effective communication (Box 6.2) that impacts on teaching, learning and self-management; remembering language includes body language, gestures and paralingual sounds that can also be different in other cultures. Technology has seen the rise of new communication methods and new words were coined to describe technology (see Chapter 12). There is some evidence that spending long periods on the Internet and email can inhibit people's ability to interpret body language (Chapter 3).

Significantly, as the title of the chapter suggests, communication problems occur when there are seemingly no cultural differences and the speaker and listener(s) share the same language. Some of the miscommunication might be due to:

- Incorrect assumptions about knowledge, competence, attitudes and behaviours, for example assuming a doctor or nurse who develops

> **Box 6.2   Some tips to help achieve effective communication**
>
> - Consider the information in Box 6.1
> - Look and listen before you speak to tune in to the other person' body language and word usage issues
> - Learn the individual's story, therein lies the factors that shaped who they are, who they might become and how to work with them effectively
> - Be fully present in the conversation
> - Adapt your language and education style and content to suit the individual and their particular needs at the time
> - Avoid discriminatory language. Reflect on the information in the DA Position Statement
> - Be knowledgeable. People with diabetes expect diabetes educators to have a broad body of knowledge about the subject but they appreciate honesty. If you do not know the answer, say so and indicate you will find out or tell the person where they can find reliable information
> - Clarify your interpretation of the individual's body language, stories and questions
> - Do not interrupt the individual when they are speaking
> - Reflect on your communication and teaching style after each encounter. What worked well? What words/phrases/metaphors/ pictures were unclear? What did you learn from the encounter that could help you do better next time?
>
> Read widely, not only diabetes-related facts. People with diabetes collect information about diabetes from many sources including friends and family, social media, movies, television programmes and advertisements, books and magazines. Educators can gain very significant insight from reading fiction and people's accounts of illness, movies and plays. Reading can enhance the educator's language skills and social and emotional intelligence.

diabetes 'knows all about it'. They might (or might not) be fluent in the biomedical diabetes dialect but have no experience of the psychosocial components.

- The way information is structured.
- How the speaker signals connections among the pieces of information.
- Whether the information flows logically.
- How the components of language are used together (Roberts 2000).

Apart from the components of speech, most of these issues also apply to written information. Great care should be taken selecting pictures. Consider the many information leaflets that adorn every diabetes educator's office. Have a look at the pictures of disembodied eyes, heart and kidneys and feet. Are they in context?

Exchanging information: a complex process

In a broad sense, communication involves exchanging representations between two often diversely different 'information-processing devices': diabetes educators and people with diabetes. Krauss and Fussell (1996) described four models of interpersonal communication: encoding/decoding, intentionalist, perspective-taking and dialogic methods.

Encoding and decoding

Encoding: the speaker conveys information using codes and signals (language) that enable information to be transmitted (encoded). The listener then decodes and interprets the information. It is easy to see how the same message can be interpreted in different ways. There is evidence that speakers try to adapt their language to the people they communicate with (Krauss and Fussell 1996). Significantly, listeners have to decode body and paralingual language well as words derive meaning from the encounter.

Intentionalist

Intentionalist refers to the difference between the literal and non-literal meaning of information. Speakers select words, metaphors and speech forms to convey information.

Perspective-taking

People's perspectives often differ; listeners may interpret information differently from the intended meaning. Thus, speakers need to try to understand and consider the listener's perspectives when selecting and formulating language/information. Perspective-taking is accomplished by two simultaneously operating processes: heuristics and information the listener gleaned during the interaction, which is influenced by the amount and responsiveness that exists within the interaction. Seeking feedback and clarifying are important strategies to achieve mutual understanding.

Dialogic

Communication is a process where the speaker and listener work collaboratively to produce shared meaning. Appropriate questions and responses are essential to arriving at a shared meaning and are more likely to occur in a therapeutic, trusting relationship. The latter is the ideal method to achieve effective person-centred diabetes education likely to lead to empowerment.

There is clear evidence that language affects a number of aspects of cognition (Hardin and Banaji 1993). These cognition aspects include:

- Visual scanning: the way a person usually reads influences their preferred direction of visual scanning.
- Verbal learning: the sound of words can affect verbal learning. For example, woman and lady might have different meanings.
- Visual memory: the way a visual stimulus is labelled can affect the way it is stored in memory. Verbalising a visual memory can produce a biased representation that can affect the application of the visual memory.
- Decision-making: the way a decision, goal or problem is worded can affect subsequent decisions.
- Problem-solving: language can facilitate or hinder problem-solving.

Language and attitude change

Aristotle pointed out in *The Rhetorica* that the appropriateness of language is 'one thing that makes people believe in the truth of your story'. He also indicated the speaker's personal character is important to their credibility and indicated communicators must 'know what they ought to say as well as how to say it'.

Persuasive messages that are easy to listen to and understand will have a greater effect on people's attitudes and behaviours: it is not only what you say but how you say it that is important.

'Voices'

HPs use several 'voices':

- The doctor voice when seeking information. They are also likely to speak 'biomedical diabetes' and not pay attention while the person with diabetes attempts to provide important psychosocial information. The following dialogue overheard in a diabetes clinic clearly illustrates such miscommunication. It also shows a missed learning opportunity for the doctor.

  DOCTOR: *It looks like your blood glucose has been high the last few days?*
  PERSON WITH DIABETES: *I haven't been eating, my dog is very sick.*

DOCTOR: *OK, if you haven't been eating, why are the glucoses so high?*
PERSON WITH DIABETES: *I've been too busy caring for my dog, taking her to the vet and giving her medicines.*
DOCTOR: *Sure, but what about your high blood glucose if you aren't eating. Why aren't you eating? Are you taking your medicines?*

- The educator voice when delivering health messages, which probably sounds similar to the preceding lost opportunity to 'learn at the learnable moment'.
- The fellow human voice when encouraging people to discuss their health problems, which is most likely to achieve shared understanding and meaning. It is essential to building therapeutic relationships (Chapter 3) (Cordella 2004).

Diabetes education often occurs in high stress situations, which can influence the voice the educator uses, particularly when both parties are stressed.

Narrative medicine

Narrative medicine is a distinct and important mode of thought and way of working with 'patients' (Charon 2008). It involves using people's illness stories and usual health care to understand, diagnose and manage the illness. People's stories can be interpreted the same way as other literary texts. Two very moving illness stories are *The Diving Bell and the Butterfly* (Bauby 1997) and *The Sound of a Wild Snail Eating* (Bailey 2011). The former is an excellent story about communicating without words and without most of the other components of speech. Both attest to the power of personal writing to transformation.

Narrative medicine is highly relevant to diabetes education and can strengthen the educator–person with diabetes relationship and is more likely to achieve person-centred care. Benefits to the educator include enhanced empathy and job satisfaction.

The value of reading fiction

In the last 25 years, psychologists have researched the importance of reading fiction to social intelligence. Stories are a type of simulation that helps readers understand the characters in the book, their relationships and social situations and human characters generally (Oatley 2011).

Reading fiction improves people's social skills, builds empathy and the ability to see other people's point of view; that is, it hones people's social brain (Oatley 2011). For example, research suggests people who read creative writing (stories) perform better on social reasoning tests than people who read the same information in a non-fiction format (Mar et al. 2009). Mar et al. (2009) suggested fiction primes people to think about the social world more sympathetically than those who do not read fiction, and fiction readers are better able to develop a theory of mind.

Theory of mind refers to the ability to understand the perspectives of other people to develop mental models of others and appreciate that people have attitudes, beliefs and intentions different from one's own. A well-developed theory of mind depends on good social skills. The development of a theory of mind starts early, about 4 years of age, and continues to develop throughout life. The more fiction people read, the more they are able to make mental models of other people (Djikic et al. 2009).

Djikic et al. found a significant association between empathic ability and fiction reader's theory of mind compared with people who did not read fiction. Interestingly, the same might not apply to watching TV, possibly because TV shows do not explore as many themes that require viewers to adopt a character's point of view (Mar et al. 2009).

MRI images suggest the reader's brain responds to fiction the same way a character in a story would react. For example, the prefrontal cortex (concerned with goal-setting) reacts when a character in a book sets a new goal. Other parts of the brain react to different situations (Speer et al. 2009).

Some chapters in this book provide examples of how stories affected the authors' thinking and ways of working that they translated into their diabetes education role. Likewise, there is a list of recommended reading and movies in Appendix, which is almost all fiction or people's illness stories. It is very difficult to decide what to include in such a list; thus, it is by no means complete and is decidedly biased by the kind of books I like. Educators can also use writing as a counselling tool.

Using writing in diabetes care

Apollo was the Greek god of poetry and medicine, and poetry was originally considered the most prestigious of the two. The relative rank has changed, but both still depend on close observation and careful use of language. In Germany, poets are regarded as the condensers or concentrators of language and metaphor because they pack the greatest amount of meaning into small linguistic spaces. Japanese haiku is an excellent example of using few words for maximum meaning.

Some people find writing a useful way of working through experiences and coming to terms with life events, especially painful negative events (Gaschler 2007; Dunning 2008). Some people feel better mentally and physically and more in charge when they write their stories than during counselling (Zable 2011).

In addition, expressive writing has a favourable influence on the immune system and blood pressure in the long term (Gaschler 2007). Some researchers suggest positive effects are more likely when people write about negative situations they have not discussed with anybody before, but recent research suggests this might not be the case. Expressive writing can be painful, but it enables people to analyse the situation and some people have been able to achieve new meaning and a more positive outlook after very traumatic events.

The following anecdote explains how/why I first began to use stories and writing with people with diabetes in the early 1980s. One of the first people I ever 'educated', educated me.

Mrs T was in her 50s: she had long standing T2DM, significant complications, and depression. She needed to commence insulin. It took a long time to establish a trusting relationship with her. She attended appointments but left if she was scheduled to see a male health professional and would not discuss her diabetes or personal situation. She had clearly not started taking her insulin because her blood glucose levels were averaging 20 mmol/L and her HbA$_{1c}$ was still 13.7%. I felt helpless and did not know how to help her.

One day I received a very thick letter from Mrs T that explained her story starting from childhood to the present situation where she was living in a park. The letter was obviously very difficult for her to write. It explained why she was not using her insulin and her attitudes to men, her several attempts at suicide and her deplorable social situation. She explained her priest and I were the only people she felt she could trust.

I was overwhelmed and humbled. Knowing her story helped me understand the low priority she placed on her diabetes, even her life, and her lack of self-esteem. I did not feel I had done anything to gain her trust or that I was equal to the challenge of helping her. From then on she visited me every week but always sent a letter first, that flagged the issues she wanted to discuss at the next visit.

Writing can be a very useful reflective process for diabetes educators too and has the same benefits as for patients.

Who is he?
I shuffled through the pieces of his life trying to make a pattern
from the stark fragments scrawled in his medical record.
Trying to see the man in the biochemistry, the catalogue of ailments,
and lists of medicines, some scratched out; others added.
I tried to link the disjointed fragments to see the whole.
The note on his door said he likes reading.
There are no books in his room.

Dunning (2009, unpublished
reflective journal)

Education materials

Most diabetes education material represent HPs (Wolpert and Anserson 2001) and often pharmaceutical company perspectives about diabetes pathophysiology, glycaemic control, lifestyle factors, medicines and long-term complications. Many people are concerned about other life priorities, understanding what the information means to their personal situation and how they can fit diabetes self-management tasks into their lifestyle. That is, they want personalised information.

The International Alliance of Patients' Organisations (IAPO) indicates HPs must recognise that many people are experts in their disease and that the content and how it is communicated needs to be considered. IAPO made a series of recommendations in a policy statement: IAPO Policy Statement on Patient Information (2005) as well as producing a number of other useful documents about engaging with patients that can be accessed from www.patientorganizations.org. It is interesting to note that IAPO uses the term 'patient', which is discouraged in the DA language Position Statement as being disempowering.

Basically IAPO, and many experts, recommend:

- Having a clear understandable message
- Using relevant and tailored content
- Using a culturally and linguistically relevant writing style and format
- Involving readers, listeners, viewers when using information
- Pilot testing with key stakeholders

I suggest it is important to involve key stakeholders in developing and testing the material, as well as cognitive debriefing to determine face and content validity. A number of tools can be used to assess literacy and the numeracy level of written material, see Chapter 10. SAM, Suitability Assessment of Materials (2008) is also useful. However, determining the literacy level of spoken language is more complex and needs to occur within the conversation. It is even more challenging in group education.

Winnie the Pooh has the last word

Winnie the Pooh's conversation with Owl clearly illustrates the importance of knowledge and experience but shows people do not necessarily speak the same language, even when they do! The scholars Winnie refers to could be diabetes educators, other HPs or academics who do not 'live in the real world' of the person with diabetes.

WINNIE: *Now one rather annoying thing about scholars is they are always using BIG WORDS that some of us can't understand ... and sometimes one gets the impression that those intimidating words are there to keep us from under-standing. That way, the scholars can appear Superior, and will not likely be suspected of Not Knowing Something. After all, from the scholarly point of view, it's practically a crime not to know everything. But sometimes the knowledge of the scholar is a bit hard to understand because it doesn't seem to match up with our own experience of things.*

OWL: *In other words, Knowledge and Experience do not necessarily speak the same language. But isn't the knowledge that comes from experience more valuable than the knowledge that doesn't?*

WINNIE: *It seems to me scholars need to go outside and sniff around—walk through the grass, talk to the animals. That sort of thing.*

Hoff (2002)

Reflective questions

Reflection is essential to learning. It is a key part of the person with diabetes' journey and it is equally important for HPs to reflect on their journey as carers and educators. The following statements or questions may help you reflect. It sometimes helps if you think about a recent encounter with a person with diabetes where you felt the encounter did not go as well as you would like.

- Reflect on Winnie the Pooh's comments. What did you learn from Winnie's point of view that applies to diabetes education?
- What kind of language would you use if you had to teach Winnie about diabetes?
- What do you think about using writing to help people with diabetes think about and manage their diabetes?
- Have you ever thought about what you can learn from reading fiction?

References

Aristotle. (1954) *The Rhetoric and the Poetics of Aristotle*. Translated by Roberts W. New York, Modern Library.

Bailey E. (2011) *The Sound of a Wild Snail Eating*. Melbourne, Victoria, Australia, Text Publishing.

Bauby J-D. (1997) *The Diving Bell and the Butterfly*. New York, Knopf Doubleday.

Bennett A. (2007) *The Uncommon Reader*. London, Faber & Faber.

Boroditsky L. (2003) Linguistic relativity. In Nadel L. (ed.), *Encyclopedia of Cognitive Science*. London, MacMillan, pp. 917–921.

Charon R. (2008) *Narrative Medicine: Honoring the Stories in Medicine*. Oxford, Oxford University Press.

Chickman I, Howett D. (2006) *Beowulf: A Dual-Language Edition*. New York, Anchor Books.

Cordella M. (2004) *The Dynamic Consultation. A Discourse Analytical Study of Doctor–Patient Communication*. Amsterdam/Philadelphia, John Benjamins.

Darwin C. (1871) *The Descent of Man*. London, John Murray Publishers.

Deutscher G. (2010) *Through the Language Glass: Why the World Looks Different in Other Languages*. London, Arrow Books.

Diabetes Australia. (2011) *A New Language for Diabetes: Improving Communication with and about People with Diabetes*. Canberra, Australian Capital Territory, Australia, Diabetes Australia.

Djikic M, Oatley K, Zoesterman Z, Peterson J. (2009) On being moved by art: How reading fiction transforms the self. *Creativity Research Journal* 21(1): 24–29.

Dunning T. (2009) Creative writing: A useful therapeutic tool. *The Art of Healing* 1(22):24–26.

Eggert M. (2010) *Brilliant Body Language*. Edinburgh, Pearson Education.

Ekman P. (1982) *Emotion in the Human Face*, 2nd edn. New York, Cambridge University Press.

Erard M. (2008) English as she will be spoke. *New Scientist* 29 March:28–32.

Flores G, Rabke-Verani B, Pine W, Sabharwl A. (2002) The importance of cultural and linguistic issues in the emergency care of children. *Paediatric Emergency Care* 18:271–284.

Frank W. (1995) *The Wounded Storyteller: Body, Illness, and Ethics*. Chicago, IL, University of Chicago Press.

Gaschler K. (2007) The power of the pen. *Scientific American Mind* August/September:14–15.

Hoff B. (2002) *The Tao of Pooh and the Te of Piglet*. London, Egmont, pp. 40 and 41.

Johnson E. (2011) Social networks matter: Friends increase the size of your brain. *Scientific American* 17 November.

Krauss R, Chiu C-Y. (1997) Language and social behaviour. In Fiske G. and Lindsey G. (eds.), *Handbook of Social Psychology*. Boston, MA, McGraw-Hill, pp. 41–88.

Lakin J. (2003) The chameleon effect of social glue. *Journal of Nonverbal Behaviour* 27:145–162.

Mar R, Oatley K, Peterson J. (2009) Exploring the link between reading fiction and empathy: Ruling out individual differences and examining outcomes. *Communications: The European Journal of Communication Research* 34(4): 407–428.

Mehrabian A. (1971) *Silent Messages Implicit: Communication of Emotions and Attitudes*, 2nd edn. Belmont, CA, Wadsworth.

My Fair Lady. (1964) Adapted from Lerner and Lowe's. Stage play by MGM pictures.

Oatley K. (2011) In the minds of others. *Scientific American Mind* November/December:63–67.

Roberts C. (2000) Professional gatekeeping in intercultural encounters. In Coulthard M. (ed.), *Discourse and Social Life*. London, Longman Pearson.

Ryback T. (2009) *Hitler's Private Library: The Books that Shaped His Life*. London, Bodley Head.

SAM Suitability Assessment of Material. (2008) Fro evaluation of health-related information for adults.

Scheeres H, Slade D, Manidis M, McGregor J, Matthiessen C. (2008) Communicating hospital emergency departments. *Prospect* 23(2):13–22.

The International Alliance of Patients' Organisations (IAPO). (2005) IAPO Policy Statement on Patient Information. www.patientorganizations.org (accessed October 2011).

Quiller-Couch C. (1916) Interlude on Jargon. *The Art of Writing, Section V.* Cambridge, Cambridge University Press.

Watson D. (2004) *Watson's Dictionary of Weasel Words, Contemporary Clichés, cant and Management Jargon.* Milson's Point, Random House.

Whorf B. (1956) *Language Thought and Reality: Selected Writings of Benjamin Lee Whorf.* Boston, MA, MIT Press.

William L, Fowler HW, Jessie C. (1973) *The Shorter Oxford Dictionary on Historical Principles Volume 1: A–Markworthy.* Oxford, Clarendon Press, p. 1174.

Willis J, Todorov A. (2006) First impressions: Making up your mind after 100 ms of exposure to a face. *Psychological Science* 17:592–598.

Wolpert H, Anderson B. (2001) Management of diabetes: Are doctors framing the benefits from the wrong perspective? *British Medical Journal* 323(7319): 994–996.

Zable A. (2011) Universal truths. *Australian Author* September:24–26.

7 Role and Use of Creative Arts in Diabetes Care

Jean-Philippe Assal and Tisiana Assal

Foundation for Research and Training in Patient Education, Geneva, Switzerland

> *Art does not reproduce the visible, but makes visible.*
> Paul Klee

Introduction

Concepts and techniques which belong to the world of art are not obvious even in medical practice. They may hurt certain aspects of the medical identity. But having experienced this unique help which the arts can offer to the quality of long-term care, physicians and other health professionals (HPs) are discovering a new dimension in their profession.

Medical identity

Doctors are trained to diagnose: and analysis what is not functioning in the human body. They act like an accountant trained to evaluate the pluses and minuses of a budget. Their role is to scan the excess expenditure, find errors in management and suggest solutions.

The same is true for HP at the time of diagnosis, in particular for emergencies. But with chronic diseases the HPs have also to accompany their patient over time. In this situation they have to adopt quite a different role. They need new skills to deal with the psychological suffering of patients in order to help them to express their difficulties in coping, doubts about healing, beliefs about the efficacy and the cost of treatment. Helping a person express their feelings is a major responsibility for all HPs involved in the accompaniment of patients suffering from chronic diseases.

Artists are accustomed to expressing and illustrating sorrow, doubts, joy, anxiety, loneliness, depression and the fear of death. The arts offer

Diabetes Education: Art, Science and Evidence, First Edition. Edited by Trisha Dunning AM.
© 2013 John Wiley & Sons, Ltd. Published 2013 by John Wiley & Sons, Ltd.

people a testimony to man's condition. Since suffering is normally endured in silence, the arts represent a unique way for people to exchange and express feelings in a metaphoric way through music, painting, writing and theatre.

The four cardinal axes of healthcare delivery

Healthcare delivery is quite a complex activity particularly for those who have to treat and accompany patients suffering from chronic diseases for several years. According to the World Health Organisation (WHO), more than 100 different diseases are listed as chronic diseases, i.e. diseases that cannot be cured but can be treated effectively if patients have been taught how to manage their own treatment. The term 'patient education' has, therefore, been replaced by Therapeutic Patient Education (TPE) in order to stress that this type of education is directly linked to its effect on the management of the disease and should be provided by HPs: doctors, nurses, nutritionists, and psychologists.

Four dimensions should be mentioned. They are medical, psychological, educational and the accompaniment dimensions. In healthcare delivery, these are constantly linked together. In integrated care none of them is ever independent from the others. It is important to grasp that there is a permanent gap between patients and caregivers. One is looking for help, the other is an "expert" at establishing diagnoses and providing the appropriate care. Great effort is made to develop a more equal relationship between both partners but there is always an imbalance between the expectations of the patient and the expertise of the caregiver.

A fundamental characteristic of chronic diseases is their duration, and the obligation of caregivers to accompany the same patient for many months or years. This situation carries risks: monotony, weariness and even burnout of all involved—the patient and their family, and all the members of the healthcare team. This is where creativity offers a unique source of renewal. Creativity offers a neutral space where the patient does not have to justify their expectations and where the caregiver may leave off their professional identity for a brief period. Both may express, through the medium of painting, theatre, music and dance, personal experiences that they may never have talked about and which may be important for their identity and the quality of their subsequent treatment.

The disease

The basics of medical education imply knowing the causes of diseases, the diagnostic procedures and the appropriate therapeutic measures to initiate. It is an important mass of theoretical knowledge and of practical experience to master. Medical activity is often bound up with an emergency. Often the very first activities of HPs are subject to the dimension of urgency. Professional identity is often shaped by first medical experiences where the patient is thankful because their pain has disappeared and that HPs know how to cure the disease.

However, more than 85% of medical visits concern chronic conditions where HPs have to change their focus from an emergency situation to a person suffering. How is the patient coping with the difficulty of not being cured? This situation requires HPs to change their approach radically and accept without frustration to accompany their patient rather than necessarily to cure him.

Understanding the clinical relationship between an HP and the patient

How many patients have been shocked by the way the diagnosis was given to them, or how little the HP realises the effects they have on their patient. Medical responsibility in biomedicine depends on rigorous diagnostic procedures and precise therapeutic choices. But medical responsibility is also a human responsibility that includes respect and solicitude towards the patient. Dealing with a chronically ill patient requires the HP to spare sufficient time to create a trustful relationship where concern is given to the way the patient copes with his disease and his illness. In this perspective, the patient becomes the subject and not the object of the concern and activity of the HP.

The therapeutic education of the patient and their family

I remember a patient who thanked me because I 'cured' him. He had diabetes and had been on insulin for 30 years. I could not understand what he meant since this type of diabetes is a lifelong condition. But this patient had intuitively sensed the role and effect of therapeutic education. Thanks to the process of education, he gradually experienced how he could manage his treatment and adapt it to his various daily activities. His success in this respect illustrates the profound effects of therapeutic education: to allow the patient to feel in control of his diabetes. He was cured of the blind passive dependence on his doctor. He discovered his own power in managing his diabetes.

The accompaniment of the patient over months and years

Solitude, loss of self-esteem and difficulty in making plans is found in almost all patients suffering from a chronic disease. One may define the chronic patient as the bearer of a heavy psychological load that they carry in silence day-after-day.

Suffering is rarely openly expressed, and if clinicians are not aware of it, it is often detected too late. Creativity and artistic expression may be a unique opportunity to help patients express their psychological reactions to their disease and help HPs to understand more about their patient and to be closer to them.

Listening to patients and modes of self-expression

There is an urgent need to promote activities where carers and patients can share some of their life experiences. There are various ways of doing this:

- Active listening
- Patient narratives about signs and symptoms of the disease and/or illness, their daily family, professional and social lives
- Painting workshops as a developmental process stimulating self-expression
- The theatre of lived experience, an opening up of the psychosocial dimension of each individual.

Promoting creativity

The direct description of true, real suffering is almost impossible. First because pain is an eminently personal experience and its direct verbal description may not be sensed correctly by the person to whom the victim addresses the description. Using the metaphor of the brightness of the sun, we cannot describe its strength in simple words. But poets can, as well as actors, artists and musicians.

The 10 year experience at our foundation has shown that an artist is hidden in each individual, even in the most sceptical. Through painting, writing, theatre and dance personal experiences can be expressed, irrespective of the cultural origin and the social background of the individual.

Painting as a process of transformation

The purpose of this chapter is to describe the structure of painting workshops and the specific benefits the participants acquire through their experience of painting. Painting workshops for people suffering from chronic conditions opened in Geneva (Switzerland) in 2004, sponsored by the Foundation for Research and training in Patient Education. At the time of writing, 50 painting workshops have been organised and 90 people have participated. In order to better understand the ability of painting to play a role in the healing process, we have looked at how artists themselves explain their own experience of painting and the painting process in general.

Structure of the painting workshop

Each painting workshop, conceived as a unit, lasts two and a half days and takes place once a month. The participants are adults suffering from a chronic condition: diabetes, obesity, anorexia, cancer, alcoholism, leg amputation or recurring depression. Groups may be heterogeneous regarding age, sex, motivation, artistic training and medical conditions or, on request, the workshop brings together homogeneous groups and focuses on specific goals.

The mean age is 50. The participants do not need to have previous experience or skill in art. The workshop size is limited to eight participants. They can arrange their particular programme following their needs: they can choose the time and frequency of sessions, the artist and the group. They can attend painting workshops as many times as they wish. Many people come on a regular basis and intensify the frequency in periods of stress. The average attendance is five times.

The teacher is a professional painter, not an art-therapist. The artist knows by experience the steps leading to creation and has a deep expertise of artistic techniques which allows them to guide the participant away from stereotypes, thus encouraging the emergence of a personal style. Artists are inclined to push the participants to experiment, to explore, to go beyond their limits and to clarify what they really want to express.

At the end of each session there is a round-table discussion of all the paintings produced. The group listens to the stories behind the paintings as told by each participant, sharing experiences and emotions. Verbalising the experience lived through helps participants understand themselves better as well as share the experience with others. 'The affective dimension of the group allowed me to feel connected again with a social life' one participant said. The heterogeneity of the group is positive: the confrontation of differences stimulates interaction and questioning about other ways of perceiving and thinking. During this round-table discussion, a group moderator favours interactions, regulates confrontations and collects data in order to evaluate the efficacy of the work done.

Results

Attending one or several workshops, the participants undergo beneficial changes in their attitudes to their condition. Let us look at three cases to see how the process of creation helped a particular individual to come to terms with their condition.

The process of creation as it has been explained by some professional painters:

The process of creation, which these three people went through, had its therapeutic effect because of the specific characteristics of the creative dynamic itself. Let us look at how various painters described it. We will see that the testimonies of our workshop participants are full of echoes of what the artists say.

Case 1

A woman, aged 45, with lung cancer, undergoing chemotherapy treatment came to the workshop in a state of deep anxiety.

She began by painting a swan and went through a very long elaboration of the picture, changing many times the size, shape and colour of the bird and of the environment. It was evident that she needed to find a picture expressing very strong personal emotions. Afterwards, during the discussion, the woman said she had painted a dream she had had. In fact the image is very dreamlike: the blue swan appears like a vision in a blue unrealistic space where the border between earth and sky has disappeared.

The woman later wrote a short story about the swan and herself. In the story, the swan was an image she had from her childhood when she lived by a lake and now she was recalling him and asking him to stay close to her. This image, charged with personal emotions, gave her a strong support in this difficult phase of her life.

Case 2

A man, aged 55, undergoing a deep depression, came to the workshop for the first time not knowing what to expect.

He was asked to paint a landscape and he did it with very pale colours. The teacher invited him to put some life in it, for instance a strong animal, maybe a buffalo. The man did it, but the buffalo, dwarfed by the mountain range, was too far away. The teacher pushed him to try new paintings of strong buffaloes, adding that in order to give the buffalo strength and credibility he had to feel in himself the aggressiveness of the buffalo. After several attempts the man came up with a strong image, and then inserted other buffaloes and finally he covered one entire wall with buffaloes fighting. At the end of the day he left the workshop as if he had fought all these terrific battles himself. He said he was feeling much better: he had really experienced the buffalo's strength.

Creation involves introspection

Matisse said every authentic effort of creation was interior (Henri Matisse 1949 in Fourcade 1992, p. 322) suggested painting has its roots in memory, more than in visual perception. Immersed in his inner world, the painter encounters and awakens old feelings and memories that have been denied or repressed and in letting them emerge he is confronted with himself. He discovers himself (Fabienne Verdier, in Charles Juillet 2007, p. 33).

Case 3

A young woman, aged 24, came to the workshop for the second time. She had diabetes from the age of 14 and had been suffering from severe anorexia in the last 5 years after a broken love relationship.

She began the workshop by painting a compact chain of mountains that immediately she felt as too oppressive. How to put a distance between that suffocating wall and herself? The artist-teacher suggested drawing a window in front of the landscape. She outdid his advice and built a real window of cardboard which she was able to open and close. It was a laborious task for her, done with deep concentration and emotion.

She then painted two separate figures, a boy and a girl waving good-bye to each other. She placed the boy near the mountains, the girl before the window and then, after some hesitation, she closed the window. She had put on a stage all the elements of her story, in a perspective under-lining the distance between each one. She had given the painting an order which was meaningful to her and she looked at the end very satis-fied and relieved. This young woman, who came frequently to the paint-ing workshops, had significant improvements in her health condition and quality of life.

In the three cases described, creation allowed the participants to get in touch with their inner feelings and express, through metaphoric images, emotions that they were not able to verbalise. They got a better understanding of themselves in this process of bringing unconscious feelings into consciousness and an increased sense of power over their condition. This is particularly true in case 1: the woman discovered in herself the permanence of an image linked to her childhood, and that image, which she painted, became like a talisman helping her through a crisis.

Transforming his inner world into pictorial metaphors, the painter generates new meanings and ways of self-awareness. One participant said: 'Those workshops have allowed me to go into the depths of myself and to understand the origin of some of my attitudes'.

Creation reactivates emotions

Matisse also emphasised that the work of art only fully existed when it was loaded with human emotion (Henri Matisse 1952 in Fourcade 1992, p. 57). In any kind of representation, one must not merely copy or follow pictorial conventions but must transform reality, projecting personal feelings and emotions into it. During the intense effort of creation, emotions take root progressively, changing, deepening, guiding.

Immersed in the emotional experience of the universe he is painting, the artist enlarges his perceptions, discovers and transforms himself while transmitting his feelings to the painting in progress, as expressed in case 2. To reactivate the world of emotions and sensitivity is very important for people with a chronic disease often weighed down by their suffering. One participant said: 'Through these workshops I have learnt to express what I feel, which was very difficult for me before'.

Creation means exploring the new and the unknown

In Picasso's view, painting means to experiment and to go through the process of continuous transformation of the work in progress. For him, changes are produced not by preparatory sketches, but by variants on the theme of that particular painting (Pablo Picasso, in Arnheim 1964, p. 22). The painter discovers his own work while he is creating it, step-by-step, changing over and over its forms and meanings. Painting appears as an experience which opens the way to new forms of thinking and this is particularly important for patients living a chronic condition, seeking a new perspective on their lives.

A participant put it: 'I discovered I can do things differently. This gives me the courage to venture off the beaten track onto other paths. This workshop has opened new horizons for me'.

Creation involves fighting against difficulties

Bacon told an interviewer that when he began a new picture, he had a certain idea of what he wanted to do, but while he was painting, suddenly, from the pictorial material itself, shapes and directions somehow came out that he had not anticipated (Francis Bacon, in Archimbaud 1996, p. 67).

As soon as the picture begins to exist, it leads the artist along unexpected paths. The process of creation leads to the realisation of the work demands, a struggle to impose order on the chaos of his feelings, and to clarify what he wants to express. Matisse saw creation as the act of putting order into chaos (Fourcade 1992). The artist and the painting in progress build each other in a game of confrontations.

It is in his relationship with the resistance of the work that the artist becomes aware of himself, clarifies his purpose and gains proof of his courage to impose himself.

One participant said a short time after the workshop: 'I was amased at what I had achieved. Painting allowed me to have another way of thinking about myself. Now I feel more secure, confident and I dare to show myself as I am'.

The painters' observations point to the double process in the act of painting: the process that leads to the realisation of the work and the process that sends the painter back to himself. Soulage confirmed to an interviewer that the painting partly created itself but it created him at the same time (Pierre Soulage, in Le Lannou 2009, p. 141).

Encouraging results

Data were collected over a period of 6 years. Analysis of transcriptions of the group's discussions at the end of each workshop and long-term effects measured by using individual questionnaires gave insight into the process of change during the experience of painting and its effects on the quality of life of the participants. Data indicated three main kinds of benefits:

1. Greater self-esteem due to awareness of personal potential
2. A sense of autonomy gained from the experience of coping with difficulties
3. A new psychological strength brought by the support of the group.

The theatre of lived experience

Its origin

In our diabetes treatment and teaching unit for patients, we gave systematic attention to the degree of coping of all our patients. For more than 20 years, we have run weekly round tables on 'How do I live with my diabetes?' Both patients and carers participated. These round tables were much appreciated by patients, who could express their personal problems and difficulties in managing their own disease.

The exposure to patients' psychological burdens helped many HPs to improve and adapt their relationship with patients. But some problems remained: some patients were still too shy to express their difficulties and physicians did not always participate, because of other professional constraints. Often the psychologists who ran the round table and followed patients over time were somewhat distant in giving useful information about their follow-up to the rest of the team.

In 2002, we developed with Marcos Malavia, a stage director, the 'theatre of lived experience' with the aim of enabling patients and health professionals to express and share their life experiences through writing and directing short plays. Since then, more than 230 participants have taken part in this creative process: patients suffering from chronic diseases such as diabetes, obesity, kidney failure, amputation, cancer, grief due to a loss, anorexia, cardiovascular diseases, depression, etc. There was also a demand from health professionals and people involved in humanitarian activities.

Artistic expression favours communication

Artistic expression is a very strong vector for sharing one's personal life experience. It provides an environment where patients and healthcare providers can share a common ground and establish a more personal and horizontal relationship, more equal and respectful. It offers them a unique space where theatre's creative process enables them to transcend their condition and life experiences.

The exchange in 'theatre of lived experience' enables carers and humanitarians to develop an ability to observe the complexity of the life of the patient or victim and for the two to increase their feeling of responsibility. This process contributes to reinforcing the empowerment of the patients and their carers in their respective identities and roles.

Two examples

Blood glucose: a number or myself … ? Brigitte

Brigitte is a 48-year-old biology teacher in a high school. She had type 1 diabetes since the age of 22. She followed quite actively our therapeutic education programme, but in spite of this, her glycated haemoglobin remained high, nearly 9%. She described well the factors responsible for the increase of blood glucose, but paradoxically she felt quite passive in trying to modify them.

The help of a psychologist was no more successful. We proposed the theatre of lived experience but she refused. Two years later, she finally accepted and wrote a dialogue between herself (BRI) and her blood glucose (BG).

> BG: *You are again too high!*
> BRI: *Shut up! You are only a figure.*
> BG: *A figure? But you know, I am you!*
> BRI: *You are nothing else but a figure. Remember how the doctor speaks about you. You are nothing else than a number! The doctor does not need to talk to you, remember.*
> BG: *When your students lack discipline or do not want to study, you go home exhausted. I witness your stress, your tiredness which brings your sugar up. I am a little part of you!*
> BRI: *Ok, but a small part only. But me, I am still not you, not you.*
> BG: *Nevertheless we have to live together.*
> BRI: *You mean that you are my shadow. May be its true, we have to live together.*
> BG: *What about going for a walk together?*
> BRI: *All right, let's go for a walk.*

A few words about the process of staging

Brigitte put the actors on two different seats placed separately at the front of the stage. The play was not satisfactory. She then proposed the actors should sit together on a bench. No results either. The professional stage director made some proposals. In order to favour a more interactive dialogue, both should sit on separate chairs and facing each other. In this position the interaction became meaningful. But sitting on the chairs did not help to develop the process of reunion of both identities.

Brigitte proposed that both actors would walk together. A partial improvement occurred but it was only when the actors put their arms round each others' shoulders and started to walk together that the staging symbolised the integration of the blood glucose in the psychological wholeness of Brigitte's body.

After the scene was played in front of Brigitte and the six other participants, she declared how visualising on stage had helped her to realise the harmful influence of the separation between herself and her blood glucose levels. Two months later, Brigitte called us and told us that her glycated haemoglobin had fallen from 9 to 7%.

See you in 1 month...

This is the story of a physician, Dr Paul A. A banal episode, apparently. While shaving in the morning he felt by chance a small nodule close to his thyroid gland. He asked a colleague, a cousin, to remove it. The operation took place without a problem. He had an appointment in the hospital for the result of the biopsy. Dr Paul A. wrote about this visit.

He had to wait for 2 hours without information, felt very tense and hardly understood his name through the loudspeaker when he was called. When the surgeon finally arrived, he simply said:

> *Sorry, it is bad news, you have cancer, an adenocarcinoma of the thyroid. Let me sign this request for treatment in the department of cancerology. Sorry again but you will see, everything will be ok. Please call if you need help. Let us meet in two months. Ciao caro.*

He then left and Dr Paul A. was left alone.

A few words about the process of staging

Dr PA did not spontaneously propose ways to organise the scene. The professional stage director did not want to impose his way immediately, he just asked: 'What kind of atmosphere existed in the hospital?' Paul said: 'Like in other hospitals, rather cold with bare corridors'. Since the stage, like all other stages, was black, she decided to hang white sheets and to transform it into a white box. Dr. Paul agreed but wanted the door through which the surgeon was to arrive to be black.

The actor had difficulty conveying Paul's tension while waiting in the corridor. It took some time to get it right. Paul was never satisfied. It was only when music was added that he felt the adequacy between his feelings and the play. In his solitude, after the diagnosis, he wrote a text which was read from behind the scene:

> If I make it, I should change my attitude toward my patients. Life is not a game, it should be lived with responsibility directed to oneself and to others. Mistakes have to be paid for in all respects: those concerning disease and illness as well as their psychological consequences.
>
> But life is also a beautiful opportunity to create and strengthen links between people.
>
> Life experiences, even painful ones, may frequently, but not always, allow us to analyse the results and make projects accordingly, by removing the superfluous and allowing the essential to emerge. If I can overcome this cancer and cope with this tumour, I should like to try to become a better individual. The time allowed us is not infinite.
>
> (Paul A., Physician)

Structure of the theatre of lived experience

The theatre consists of a 3 day workshop that brings together about eight people in a multistage process.

Day 1: the participants write a text (dialogue or monologue) relating a significant personal experience. There is no pressure to speak about their health or professional identity (healthcare provider or humanitarian worker).

At the end of the 1st day, each participant reads his text to the group. Readings are often quite emotional, with the reader sometimes in tears.

Day 2: all the texts are read by professional actors, which offers the participants a sense of distance vis-à-vis their own text. Then each participant individually and in turn begins putting his own text on stage. He directs the actors, sets the stage, experiments with lights, chooses the music, etc. A professional stage director accompanies each participant throughout the whole process. It can take up to 3 hours to produce a short play of approximately 5 min.

Day 3: all the plays are presented as a single entity in an order chosen by the professional stage director.

The theatrical representation adds an essential element to the initial text: the words are brought to life thanks to the actors, while staging brings colour, movement and music. A past life experience can thus come back to life; through the metaphoric power of theatre, the participant can express what words alone often cannot. The theatre, as a place where words are brought to life, participates in the transformation of the life experience.

Gaining perspective

Becoming aware of others' struggle enables us to distance ourselves from our own suffering and to see it as part of a much wider picture. Consequently each participant gains access to his own creative resources and to an increased sense of power over his own condition. The theatre of lived experience provides a space where groups can express many of their feelings related to health and life in general.

Some of the reactions of patients, doctors and nurses who participated in this theatrical process:

> *At the beginning I was almost panicked, I never tried to talk about myself, it was difficult, but when I saw my colleagues in the same situation I felt somehow relieved.*

Discovering the common universal ground on which everybody stands, various participants said: 'Everyone's story becomes my own story as well'. The theatrical process enables the health professionals and the humanitarians to modify the image they have of the patient or the victim. In so doing they can demonstrate that they are more than technicians or scientists.

The stage director, the coordinator and the actors are professionals of the theatre, not directly involved in the therapy. This is an essential element for creating a neutral ground where patients and victims, healthcare providers and humanitarians can express themselves on an equal level and in a context other than the medical and humanitarian worlds. But for patients it is essential that a physician, who knows the theatrical process well, be present.

Some particular aspects

For the participants

'I never lived such an experience; everyone listened to me during these three days!' Solitude is the common denominator of all participants whether patients or healthcare providers. In the classical way of interviewing a patient about how his treatment has gone, there is a great interest in what has been achieved in a quantitative way and little interest in qualitative factors dealing with the psychosocial experience. The theatrical process tries to make up for this imbalance.

A special group dynamic occurs where we mix heterogeneity of culture and life experience. Everybody is equal in their diversity. Eating together for 3 consecutive days generates spontaneous interactions and reinforces human bonds.

For the actors

The play script is often not clear. It is not written by a professional playwright. 'As an actress at the beginning I felt frustrated by this lack of professionalism by the author, but later when I watched the work done on stage, with the efforts of the stage director, I discovered the true sense of the role', said one actor.

For the stage director

The staging helps the writer understand what the text really means. It is quite interesting to observe the expression of the author when the staging really reflects what they wanted to express. The written text may sometimes be too harsh and cruel. When the same written message is expressed on the stage, the distancing process gives the spoken words a more subtle meaning. The text acquires a life of its own.

The use of lighting and music

Like the use of lighting to create an atmosphere through its intensity and colour on stage, music may reinforce the text. I remember the story of a man who wrote a text about his father who was very demanding and imposed all sorts of rules on his children. The text was somehow banal, maybe because this man did not want to complain too much. The stage director then asked: 'What kind of music would best represent your father's character?' Several suggestions were made but they did not satisfy him. The following morning this man brought a CD *Marches of the Red Army Military Band*. It was not in words but in music that he was able to express the character of his father.

The general moderator

The moderator has a most important role to fulfil. They must have extensive training and experience in this form of theatre. They assure the links between the different specialists: from the field of theatre, medicine and the humanitarian world, and have the difficult task of ensuring that each performance is patient, or victim, centred. They have to visit future participants and have to follow them after the experience. They protect the privacy of each of them.

Key learning

The experience of the creative workshops helped the participants express their personal inner suffering and deal with the psychological burden linked to a chronic disease or to a traumatic event. By getting involved in the process of creation, the participants were able to gain new insights into their subjective experience and to discover ways of improving their quality of life. They started a process of transformation.

Painting workshops are particularly suitable for people who have difficulty verbalising their experiences and emotions. Painting creates meanings through shapes and colours. One participant, a new immigrant, knowing only a few French words, said she was surprised at how much of herself she could express with a paintbrush. Another participant, a woman who was a psychoanalyst, tried to express her experience in these terms: 'When a feeling or an idea or a dream is painted, it takes a shape, it becomes more concrete. It is there and you can look at it from the outside, from a certain distance. You get the feeling that you can control it, understand it better and you feel released.'

The theatre of lived experience acts in the same way. The medical and humanitarian worlds, the pedagogical and psychosocial worlds induce a permanent imbalance between those who act, healthcare providers and humanitarian workers, and those who need help, the patients and the victims. The separation creates a world of solitude and things left unsaid. Communication through theatre can help fill this permanent gap.

Sharing their life experiences helps health professionals and patients to find a common ground on which to meet. Art provides a space where both groups can express many of their feelings related to health, life in general and their personal life experience. In this artistic space both patients and healthcare providers have the same power and role; doctors do not need to be doctors and patients do not need to be patients. Only their life experience matters. It is in the process of verbalising silence that the theatre of lived experience builds its dynamic.

Art and therapeutic education

Living with a chronic disease, mastering the complexity of treatment is often a heavy burden. Diabetes education has shown its effect, but many health professionals often doubt its long-lasting effect. Many hope the pedagogical effect can be reinforced by creative thinking.

To approach this challenging theme, it may be useful to draw the role and functioning of our brain with its cerebral left and right hemispheres.

Optimal use of left and right cerebral hemispheres may help patients to cope with their disease. The left-brain hemisphere stimulates speech and verbal expression; it promotes the use of words and of numbers, the sense of analysis, the elaboration of lists, sequences and linear analysis. The left-brain is analytical, centred on details and used primarily at the time of school and studies.

Teaching and learning in schools of medicine and nursing depend on these functions. The diagnosis of disease relies mainly on known precise facts and lists of details. This is reinforced by a process of comparison at the time of differential diagnosis.

The right-brain hemisphere participates in the holistic and creative approach (see Chapter 6).

The right-brain favours subjective, emotional participation. This hemisphere helps to translate in an artistic and musical way the difficulties and the joy of human life. It reinforces imagination, intuitive free thinking and wholeness of the situation.

The functions of both sides of the brain are connected. Professional activities such as administration, banking, economy, truck driving, flying, etc., are mainly left-brain dependent. On the other hand, creators, painters, actors, musicians and stage directors function mainly with the right-brain hemisphere. A great painting, or a musical or theatrical interpretation, is mainly the result of the right hemisphere influence.

Teachers have the responsibility to provide information through a cognitive approach (left-brain), but the great teachers use also their creative right-brain capacity to provide students with enjoyable, memorable courses. The standing ovation of the audience is often due to the 'help' of the right hemisphere that adds interest and emotion to the knowledge provided by the left-brain.

In medicine, health professionals who work in the operating room and other surgical wards function with efficacy thanks to the various performances of their left-brain. However, those who have to accompany patients over time with, for instance, type 2 diabetes, have to rely more on their right-brain in order to motivate the people they treat to adhere to the therapeutic regimen through all sorts of creative (right-brain) processes but also cognitive skills-oriented (left-brain) approaches.

The left- and right-brain hemispheres function together in a kind of interaction.

The type of professional activity chosen may reinforce the function of the right or left hemisphere. The more the specific hemisphere is solicited, the better it may perform. This is an advantage for the performance but also a handicap for the use of the opposing other hemisphere. The duality is a real challenge for training health professionals who, during training, have focussed more on the left hemisphere. Great effort is needed to fill the gap between left and right hemispheres. One difficulty is linked to the damaging belief that the creative approach always undermines the analytical or scientific part of cognition.

Clinicians have to follow chronic patients over the years. Some treat patients suffering from crippling complications (lower extremity amputation, blindness, neuropathies, renal insufficiency). These health professionals have developed an equilibrium where they have intuitively optimalised the simultaneous role and influence of their left- and right-brain hemispheres, skills and creativity.

Using creative art as an adjunct to medical care might produce benefits through the processes identified in Table 7.1.

Table 7.1   **Some benefits of using the creative arts in diabetes education and care and the processes by which the benefits occur.**

Benefits	Processes
Reinforced self-awareness	Through the process of introspection inherent to the artistic creation
Increased self-esteem	Linked to discovery of personal potential, resources and competences
A new sense of power and self-efficacy	By learning to cope with the difficulties encountered in the process of creation
Reinforced resilience and autonomy	By encouraging new ways of perceiving negative experiences and stimulating a positive active attitude to life
Reduced sense of isolation and solitude	Coming from the group's support and interaction

Summary

HPs have to take advantage of the functions provided by the left and right hemispheres. They are different but they function in a complementary way: left versus right hemisphere, analytic versus global, logical versus intuitive, objective versus subjective, detail versus wholeness, numbers versus creation, factual versus imaginative, sequential versus random, etc. Skills acquired for the management of these two extremes may greatly help HCPs to improve their attitude and quality of care delivery to their patients, either at the time of diagnosis and emergencies, or during their accompaniment over the months or years that follow.

Taking into consideration the cognitive capacities (left-brain) and the creative resources (right-brain) of the patient provides a further holistic medical approach for the patient. How to promote the use of art to provide an environment that facilitates learning and helps to soothe patients.

Patients and HPs live in a complex society. The medical organisation, like all organisations, tries to maintain the acquired structures of health and to control as much as possible the costs of care. This left-brain machinery, due to its mode of functioning, has great difficulties in understanding the importance of including, in the care process, sectors where creativity can play an equally therapeutic role.

As we saw at the beginning of this chapter, painting workshops for patients and the theatre of lived experience demonstrated their value in soothing the burden of the disease.

It is the responsibility of senior physicians and nurses to promote such an approach and to include the help of artists whose right-brain hemisphere may offer value in terms of therapy for patients. What do HPs need to learn in order to be able to blend art and science, or right and left cerebral hemispheres? There is much literature (including e-sites) which deal with creative thinking, left and right hemisphere and the function of art in education. More than 10 years' experience in this field has shown us the limits of written documents, the danger of e-programmes which claim to reinforce personal motivation, as well as the danger of promotional marketing activities, positive thinking. HPs have to deal with patients, they have to treat the disease and also soothe the burden of the illness which should be their main ethical objective. This approach requires much personal insight, and sharing within a group the complexity of this specific issue. The biggest trees grow slowly, and the correct therapy for chronic patients requires quietness, modesty and open-minded empathetic HPs.

Reflective questions

Reflection is a key part of the person with diabetes' journey: it is equally important for HPs to reflect on their journey as an HP and educator. Following are some questions you might like to reflect on. It sometimes helps if you think about a person with diabetes you educated recently and felt you did not do the job as well as you would like to.

- Have you ever used creative art in diabetes education?
- If so, what happened?
- What did you learn about yourself?

Recommended reading

On painting workshops

Archimbaud, M. (1996) *Francis Bacon, Entretiens*. Gallimard, Paris.

Arnheim, R. (1964) *Guernica, Genesi di un Dipinto*. Feltrinelli, Milan.

Assal, T. (October 2009) Art as a development process for people with a chronic condition. *Diabetes Voice*, 54(Special issue).

Demartini, D. (2009) *Le Processus de Création Picturale*. L'Harmattan, Paris.

Fourcade, D. (1992) *Henri Matisse, Écrits et Propos sur l'art*. Hermann, Paris.

Juillet, C. (2007) *Entretien avec Fabienne Verdier*. Albin Michel, Paris.

Le Lannou, J.-M. (2009) *Pierre Soulage, Écrits et propos*. Hermann, Paris.

On theatre of lived experience

Assal, J.-P., Malavia, M., Roland, M. (2009) *De la Mise en Scène à la Mise en Sens*. L'Harmattan, Paris.

Balint, M. (1964) *The Doctor, His patient, and the Illness*. Pitman Medical, London. ISBN 0 272 79206 3.

Barabino, B., Malavia, M., Assal, J.-P. (2007) The creative elaboration of a real-life experience and its transformation in a work of art. *Journal of Medicine and the Person*, 5.

Brook, P. (1977) *The Empty Space*. Penguin Books, Harmondsworth. ISBN 0141189223.

Goleman, D. (1995) *Emotional Intelligence*. Bantam Books, New York. ISBN 0-553-09503-X.

Greenhalgh, T., Hurwitz, B. (Eds.) (2000) *Narrative Based Medicine*. BMJ Books, London. ISBN 0-7279-1223-2.

Grotowski, J., Brook, P. (1975) *Towards a Poor Theatre*. A & C Black, London. ISBN 0413349101.

Helmann, C. (2006) *Suburban Shaman. Tales from Medicine's Frontline*. Hammersmith Press, London. ISBN 1-905-14008-8.

Lacroix, A., Assal, J.-P.H. (2003) *Therapeutic Education of Patients*, 2nd edn. Maloine, Paris. ISBN 2 224 02804 0.

Lowe, S.M. (2006) *The Diary of Frida Kahlo: An Intimate Self-Portrait*. Harry N. Abrams, Inc., New York.

Moffitt, D., Brook, P. (1999) *Between Two Silences: Talking with Peter Brook*. A & C Black, London. ISBN 0413755800.

Pontalis, J.-B. (2000) *Fenêtres*. Folio Gallimard, Paris. ISBN 2-07-042157-0.

8 Turning Points and Transitions: Crises and Opportunities

Trisha Dunning AM

Deakin University and Barwon Health, Geelong, Victoria, Australia

> *Ah Love! could thou and I with Fate conspire*
> *To grasp this sorry Scheme of Things entire,*
> *Would not we shatter it to bits—and then*
> *Re-mould it nearer to the Heart's Desire!*
> Omar Khayyam (1965, Rubaiyat 73)

Introduction

Life follows a natural process of beginnings and endings, or transitions that can enhance or hinder transformation and self-growth. Most people make approximately 10–20 major transitions over their lifetime. Most transitions are triggered by a turning point or event (Sugarman 2004). The way the individual responds to the trigger is more important than the trigger itself (Rogers 1991). That is, change is neither good nor bad: the way the individual perceives the change makes it one or the other.

Adaptation to small transitions often occurs through learning: however, more significant transitions that challenge self-identity, beliefs, behaviour and hope require significant reflection, healing and adaptation. Accepting change, even positive change, healing and adapting usually takes time (Williams 1999).

Transitions are crucial opportunities for healing, self-growth and development (see Chapter 5) and self-growth is possible until the moment of death, which some people regard as the ultimate transformation. Life transitions are challenging because they force people to let go of the familiar and move into the future. Making major transitions involves grieving and follow a similar emotional roller coaster as grieving over any

Diabetes Education: Art, Science and Evidence, First Edition. Edited by Trisha Dunning AM.
© 2013 John Wiley & Sons, Ltd. Published 2013 by John Wiley & Sons, Ltd.

loss (Kubler-Ross 1969). Transitions are also part of an individual's spiritual life journey (becoming) and usually require some degree of change: although most people tend to resist change, even when the benefits are clear.

The seven ages of man

There are many psychological and philosophical theories to explain common life stages and transitions: most encompass psychological, social, spiritual and moral development from various perspectives. Many of these theories also influenced teaching, learning and health-care practices. Such life stages are often referred to as the 'ages of man'.

The 'ages of man' is a well-known theme in art and literature: but the number of 'ages' described varies, for example ancient philosophers such as Aristotle described three or four ages, while medieval philosophers usually described seven ages.

One of the best-known descriptions of the 'seven ages of man' is Jaques' monologue in Shakespeare's (1964) play *As You Like It* (Act II Scene iv), which begins:

> *First, the infant, mewling and puking in his nurse's arms*

Shakespeare then describes childhood, the lover, the soldier, the justice, old age, and finally the seventh stage, dementia and death:

> *In that second childishness and mere oblivion,*
> *Sans teeth, sans eyes, sans taste, sans everything.*

The aim of each stage is to redefine the self. Jung referred to the search for identity as 'individuation', Maslow called it 'self-actualisation' and Sheehy 'gaining authenticity'. These terms all refer to the process of defining the 'individual self', fulfilling group expectations and achieving a balance between independent creative freedom and belonging to a common group.

Common descriptions of life stages include infancy and adulthood but the stages of childhood and adolescence are perhaps better known than the stages of adulthood. The latter is the main focus of this chapter. Although people's experiences and emotional responses to life transitions are individual and personal, there are many commonalities (Erikson 1950; Williams 1999; Sheehy 1995). Erikson (1950) believed that although many personality characteristics are inborn, some are learned from the challenges and support the child receives as they mature, and significantly, the effects of culture and events in the external world such as war.

Thus, Erikson regarded development as an outcome of the interaction among genetic programming, the psyche and ethos (cultural) influences. Erikson indicated the child's world gets bigger as they grow and mature and regarded failure as the result of cumulative negative events.

In contrast, Levine (2008) regarded human development as a spiralling cycle rather than hierarchical stages that each need to be completed before the next stage begins. Likewise, some versions of Kubler-Ross' (1969) grief cycle portray the grief response as a circle consisting of various stages:

- Denial
- Anger
- Bargaining
- Depression
- Acceptance

Some later versions of the grief cycle include 'shock' as the first stage of grief and insert a 'testing' stage after the depression stage. Significantly, the grief cycle is not peculiar to death and dying: these emotional reactions apply to any bad news and loss. The diagnosis of diabetes represents bad news and loss for many people (Chapters 2 and 10) and many people with diabetes experience most, if not all the stages in Kubler-Ross' grief cycle (figure 15.1, Dunning 2009, p. 420). Others accept the diagnosis and are relieved 'it's diabetes and not something worse like cancer'.

Interestingly, life transitions are sometimes regarded as major crises. The two Chinese characters *wēi jī* are widely believed to mean danger and

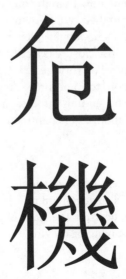

Figure 8.1 *Wēijī*, the Chinese character for crisis, with special thanks to Yen Yang for the calligraphy.

opportunity by motivational speakers, but the interpretation may not be completely accurate. *Wēi jī* does contain elements of both meanings. *Wēi* means danger or risk; *jī* has many secondary meanings including crucial point (similar to the western trigger or turning point). Linguistic experts generally agree a close approximation of the meaning is 'precarious moment' (Mair 2009); thus, the way the individual views the precarious moment and deals with the situation makes the crisis an opportunity or a threat. *Wēi jī* is shown in Figure 8.1.

Common major life transitions

A broad overview of human growth and development and the major transitions (ages and stages) are shown in Table 8.1. As indicated, the focus of this chapter is on adult life transitions. Life transitions are defined as:

> *Predictable changes in our lives associated with a discontinuity with the past. With each change we must give up the protective structures which have carried us through and then face the world anew.*
>
> Emotional Wellness Matters (1998–2004)

Bridges (1991) divided transitions into three major stages: an ending, a neutral zone and a new beginning. It is essential that people let go of the old/known in order to move on to a new beginning. New beginnings can be challenging, especially when the trigger event is unexpected and viewed as a threat or danger. Endings are difficult for most people: 'better the devil you know than the one you don't'. Some people avoid letting go by clinging to their old, known ways (denial); others dismiss the old: 'it's in the past, it's no longer relevant'. Most experts maintain it is important to let go because closure is a critical part of transformation and enables the person to move on (Bridges 1991; Sheehy 1995; Levine 2008).

In addition to the three major transitional stages, Bridges (1991) described the ending process as having four stages: disengagement, disidentification, disenchantment and disorientation.

Disengagement

Disengagement involves making a break from usual roles, activities and situations. Disengagement refers to psychological disengagement and the ability to reflect on the past objectively. It does not necessarily entail physically leaving or moving.

Disidentification

Disidentification refers to reflecting on and adjusting self-concept, for example, changing one's concept of being a younger person and accepting one

Table 8.1 **Broad stages of growth and development organised according to the primary development tasks in each stage; however, the 'boundaries' of each stage are not fixed: individual differences need to be considered.**

Life stage/transition Stages are variable but occur about every 6–10 years	Major 'tasks' associated with the stage People question and reappraise existing life structures and explore possibilities for the future
Early childhood: birth to age 8	Associated with rapid growth. The primary task is *developing skills* including fine motor skills Socioemotional development occurs at about 1 year. Thus, attachment becomes critical and the quality of the attachment can affect later relationships Cognitive development including acquiring language By 8, children have a basic understanding of some abstract concepts but still reason in a concrete way and have difficulty understanding abstract concepts
Middle childhood: 8–12	The primary development task is *integration*, within the individual and within the social context Cognitive skills, personality, motivation and inter-personal relationships develop and children learn to value society Independence increases, friendships and interests develop Skills required for academic success become more complex and challenging
Adolescence: 12–18	A diverse number of changes occur simultaneously and bring many new responsibilities and move the adolescent towards independence The primary development task is *forming an identity* Individuals develop their self-concept within their peer group. Conflict between identity and role can occur as the individual tries to match who they want to be with what is socially acceptable and meet other people's expectations Hormonal, mood changes and behaviour influence each other, fluctuate and can affect self-esteem Adolescence is usually accompanied by a growth spurt and cognitive development; but growth varies among individuals and between the genders Sexual maturation occurs during adolescence
Early adulthood: 18–30	Begin to develop meaningful relationships and their work and life path The individual can become isolated if they are unable to develop satisfying relationships with a partner and friends and may seek or avoid commitment
Mid-life: 30–40	Perplexing dissatisfaction can occur and is often associated with an event such as loss of a job or divorce, which can be a shock and triggers the need to re-authenticate self People may have outgrown some of their earlier life choices and explore neglected aspects of the self such as likes and dislikes and hobbies Ages 37–42 are peak anxiety years
40–50	'Life begins at 40' Stagnation and disequilibrium often occur in the early 40s: people ask: 'was it worth it? Is this all there is?' Mid-40s is often a period of stability and renewed purpose and independence
50–60	Often a more settled time Many people prepare to retire or retire, which might create financial constraints and new opportunities
Older age: over 60	Many people remain active but physical and mental changes become apparent Some people develop health and other problems that affect their independence Preparing for end of life care becomes more important as the person grows older Friends and relatives may die and create loneliness and stress

These definitions come from many sources; refer to Box 1. In addition to classification by age, life stages are defined culturally and socially. These ages and stages influence learning and skills acquisition. They impact on and are affected by diabetes.

has reached middle age (the mid-life crisis) or accepting oneself as a person with diabetes when the diagnosis is made (see Chapter 2). Inner conflict can occur and impede the transition process if self-concept is not adjusted.

Disenchantment

When an individual's situation and self-concept changes, they question past actions and assumptions that supported and defined the old situation, for example the belief that their marriage would 'last forever' or they would always be young and healthy.

Disorientation

Disorientation is often uncomfortable and confusing. Things that were meaningful no longer seem so important. Frankl (1969) agreed with other psychologists that biology and conditioning shape people's personalities and behaviours but maintained people were multidimensional and possessed free will (choice) to determine the meaning and purpose of their lives and take responsibility for their decisions.

Once the ending process is accomplished and the person resolves the emotional issues, they enter the neutral zone.

Neutral zone

In the neutral zone, people often take time to be alone and think, reflect and/or pray without the constraints of the old world. People often emerge from the neutral zone with new insights that prepare them for the new beginning. Thus, the neutral zone can be a time of healing and renewal in preparation for a new beginning.

A new beginning

As new information and experiences are understood and put into context, individuals develop the confidence to move on. People may seek external signs of their new beginning, but essentially the change comes from within through reflection and applying their new self-knowledge. When the new direction is clear, the new life stage begins. Significantly, new beginnings require continuity with the past because the past is a valuable knowledge store and resource for the future. Compassionate understanding of and insight into what the transition means to the individual and therapeutic support from health professionals, family and friends can enhance the likelihood the person will find meaning in the event and make a positive transition and self-growth.

As people go through the transition stages they:

- Experience a range of emotions such as loss of control, anxiety, anger, self-doubt, confusion, vulnerability and loss of self-esteem/self-image. However, the initial reaction depends on a number of factors including whether the transition is positive or negative and the individual's coping style, locus of control and resilience.
- Experience a defining moment when they begin to accept the need to change—the turning point.
- Enter a recovery phase where the individual acknowledges the need to let go of the past in order to move forward. Letting go of the past is not the same as rejecting it.
- Begin to feel hopeful and optimistic about the future, self-esteem increases and they begin to feel able to take control over the situation and the future. There is a difference between being 'in control' and controlling. The latter concerns micromanaging: being in control refers to attending to what can be done, focusing on the positive, utilising available resources and being proactive.

People move backwards and forwards through the transition stages; the transition may take some time to accomplish, often months to years. Some very poignant accounts of significant health issues clearly show the human potential to heal and that people continue to find meaning and recreate the self, even in the face of devastating disease, for example Bailey's *The Sound of a Wild Snail Eating* (2011) and Bauby's *The Diving Bell and the Butterfly* (1997), Sacks' *The Man Who Mistook His Wife for a Hat* (1985) and the movie *The Doctor* (1991) (Levinson 1978).

These stories highlight the importance of 'knowing what sort of person has a disease' (Hippocrates 460–377 BC) and could be essential reading for all health professionals.

Major life transitions

Major adult life transitions happen at roughly the same ages for all people and are associated with common feelings. Rogers (1991) suggested people should view life as a flowing process and accept themselves as a continual 'stream of becoming' rather than as an unchanging finished product. Life transitions can be key risk times for people with diabetes 'going off the rails', being 'out of control', having blood glucose 'all over the place', not undertaking appropriate self-care and hence suffering emotional distress.

These reactions suggest turning points and life transitions should be considered when taking a health and diabetes history, planning diabetes education and care, the annual complication assessment and when an individual is emotionally distressed.

Table 8.2   Major diabetes-related transitions that are superimposed on or drive usual life
transitional stages.

Diabetes-related transitions	Relationship to stages of the major life transitions
Predicaments	Normal
Diagnosis of diabetes	Ending of the old but it is common for people to deny the
Diagnosis might occur during another	diagnosis, often for a long time in an attempt to hold onto
illness, a diabetes complication or during	the old/known life
pregnancy	These factors create additional uncertainty, fear and
	vulnerability
Moving among care services, especially	Ending and a new beginning and may be neutral for
moving from child to adult care settings	some people
Commencing insulin especially for people	Often engenders fear and the need to reassess life
with type 2 diabetes	habits
Developing a complication	Loss
End of life	The ultimate transition

During life and diabetes-related transitions, unstable blood glucose levels and emotional reactions are
common and can affect self-care and coping.

In addition to life transitions and their effects on diabetes, diabetes-related transitions occur and also require the individual to reflect on and adjust to change (see Table 8.2). It can be particularly difficult for an individual with diabetes when a life transition coincides with a diabetes-related transition, which is common, for example when a woman develops gestational diabetes during pregnancy and learns she needs insulin or when an adolescent moves from paediatric diabetes services to adult services.

Transitions cause significant stress within relationships. For example, most married couples enter major life transitions such as the mid-life crisis at different times; unless they have a good relationship and communicate effectively, the marriage may not survive. Moving from paediatric to adult care is stressful for the individual and their family and often involves several simultaneous transitions, for example, leaving school, leaving home and commencing work or university.

Key transition triggers/turning points for people with diabetes include leaving school and leaving home, commencing university, graduating from university, marriage and childbirth (Rasmussen et al. 2007). Some transitions such as childbirth have sub-stages: prenatal, pregnancy, and post-natal, which have different risks and require different problem-solving and coping strategies, some of which threaten independence. Rasmussen et al. (2007) found the transition to motherhood triggered a guilt dynamic between mothers and daughters that caused them stress and to question themselves, which had not been recognised previously.

Sometimes people do not make successful transitions—they remain 'stuck' often in the ending stage and are unable to move on. Some people want to stay within the security of the known, for example people with type 2 diabetes often try to avoid commencing insulin:

No matter what I do I cannot get my blood levels [glucose] *down. Now the doctor is saying I am not eating the right things and I have to do exercise or he will put me on insulin. That is the last straw—the failure straw. I am trying to look after my wife since her stroke I can't start insulin now.*

The degree of support and quality of the relationships available to the individual and their sense of personal control over the situation have a significant effect on the transition process, but ultimately the transition and related decisions are the individual's responsibility. As Dr Seuss said:

You have brains in your head.
You have feet in your shoes.
You can steer yourself any direction you choose.
You're on your own, and you know what you know.
And you are the only one who'll decide where you'll go.
(Dr Seuss 1990)

Signs a person may be entering or is in a life transition

People respond differently to major crises but there are some common behaviours that could indicate an individual is entering a major transition. These include:

1. Mood swings—highs and lows
2. Feeling impatient or discontented with their current situation
3. Unhappiness, emotional distress or depression
4. Changed interests, hobbies taking up new ideas
5. Substance abuse such as alcohol, taking up smoking again after quitting and illegal drugs
6. Diabetes-related indicators include:
   a. Unstable blood glucose pattern
   b. Change from not attending to diabetes self-management to undertaking self-management or vice versa
   c. Not attending appointments
   d. Not taking medicines
   e. Not monitoring blood glucose

Strategies to help people manage life transitions

Skinner (1971) indicated people change their behaviours according to what they learn to ensure their survival (or not) and act according to what reinforces their actions. In order to understand why people act the way they do, health professionals need to understand the circumstances that led to their choices and actions, that is the total situation.

Before I treat a patient like yourself I need to know a great deal more about him than the patient can always tell me. Indeed, it is often the case that my patients are only pieces of a total situation, which I have to explore. The single patient who is ill by himself, is rather the exception.

Eliot (1950)

A key role for health professionals is to understand the total situation and help people with diabetes make sense of their life experiences so they can manage life's challenges and achieve social coherence (Antonovsky 1979 and 1987). Antonovsky described three essential aspects of social coherence. The three aspects are comprehensibility (cognitive), manageability (behaviour) and meaningfulness (motivation); however, the individual must have the required physical and mental ability and access to relevant resources to achieve social coherence.

Health professionals can help people with diabetes manage transitions by using effective communication and teaching techniques (see Chapters 3, 5 and 6), giving the message that change is a natural part of life, and grief and loss are normal reactions to significant changes and will resolve over time. As Homer (1966) said:

Bear patiently, my heart for you have suffered heavier things.

In particular, they can support the individual to:

1. Take time to reflect on and understand their previous life transitions, the current situation and their reactions because:

    Men are not worried by things, but by their ideas about things. When we meet with difficulties, become anxious or troubled, let us not blame others, but rather ourselves, that is: our ideas about things.

    (Epictetus, dates unknown)

2. Develop a 'life line' of previous good and not so good transitions to gain perspectives about their life course and emotional history and the coping strategies that were effective or not effective (Eos 1997–2001). Photograph albums, diaries and journals also provide information about an individual's life journey and can be very useful in aged care settings. Stout (2009) developed a useful pro forma for recording important information.

3. Think about supportive relationships, coping strategies and problem-solving methods that comfort them and make them feel secure.

4. Find answers for themselves, rather than telling the individual how they should feel or act. It is the individual transition; they need to be supported to take control and manage it and be responsible for their decisions.

5. Accept the self: talents, foibles, fears, worries that make up the individual's character, and influences how they cope with transitions. Questions to help the individual reflect include:
    a. What do you think about the situation?
    b. What do you like about yourself?
    c. What would you change if you could?
    d. How do you usually cope with problems?
6. Seek ways to manage discomfort, anxiety, insecurity and emotional distress, which might mean temporarily reprioritising activities and goals, but it is important to keep some things the same.
7. Take care of the physical, spiritual, psychological and emotional self. Managing stress is an important aspect of self-care. Refreshing sleep, a healthy diet and exercise are key self-care strategies. Self-care also involves psychological self-care, which might be achieved through prayer, meditation, support groups, counselling or a combination of methods. The medicine regimen may need to be adjusted to optimise glycaemic control.
8. Focus on the positive to maintain hope, for example, 'Just when the caterpillar thought the world was over he became a butterfly' (anonymous).
9. Ask for help.
10. Take one step at a time rather than making major decisions without weighing options and the risks, benefits and costs. Sometimes, sleeping on it helps (Chapter 3).
11. Build resilience (Clarke and Nicholson 2010; Marina-Tompkins 2011).
12. Proactively plan for predictable turning points and transitions such as anniversaries, holidays, moving house and travel. Strategies might include revising sick day management, learning how to manage stress, planning for end of life and preparing advanced care directives.

Health professionals can use most of these strategies to manage their own life transitions and to consider whether they could have a conflict of interest if their own transition (e.g. mid-life crisis) coincides with a person with diabetes' mid-life crisis.

Building resilience

> So long as a man imagines he cannot do this or that, so long is he determined not to do it; and consequently so long is it impossible to him that he should do it.
>
> (Spinoza 1632)

Health professionals can help people with diabetes learn from personal experience, particularly when they regard people's experiences as opportunities

Table 8.3   **The major positive and negative expected adult life transitions.**

Positive transitions	Negative transitions
Marriage	Serious illness
Having a baby	Significant losses, e.g. job/business,
Starting a career, university/college	partner, beloved pet, miscarriage
Buying a house	Moving into aged care facilities
Buying a car	Financial insecurity

Positive transitions are associated with 'gains' and maybe easier to cope with than negative transitions, which are usually associated with loss. Diabetes is usually regarded as a negative transition; but some people regard it as positive, which shows transitions can have both positive and negative elements. Life transitions can be planned or unexpected, as is usually the case with diabetes, especially type 1 diabetes.

for learning and seizing the day (*Carpe Diem*). A very memorable moment for me, and an excellent example of becoming and transformation, was when an 18-year-old girl with type 1 diabetes since age 8 who had repeated admissions for ketoacidosis and 'non-compliance' said:

> *I didn't want diabetes, and I don't like it, AND I still don't want it, but I can see now that diabetes helps me be who I am.*

Dilts (1990) developed the Logical Levels Model as a way of helping the individual analyse their situation and plan how to address it. The Logical Levels Model encompasses all of the factors in Antonovsky's (1979) social coherence theory discussed earlier in the chapter. The Logical Levels Model consists of five levels:

1. Environment, which refers to anything in the external environment including other people's behaviour.
2. Behaviours, those individual aspects other people see.
3. Capability, the individual's knowledge and skills.
4. Beliefs and values, the way the individual views the world and the factors that motive them.
5. Identity, the self (who am I?).

Ecomaps (Dunning 20090, p. 39) and the arts (Chapter 7) can also elicit important information about the individual's relationships and environment that can help identify supportive and unsupportive relationships. Objectively examining these issues can help the individual and the health professional determine how to enhance resilience. Although some people are more resilient than others, people respond differently to different events and have individual 'tipping points'.

Traits that promote or reduce resilience are shown in Table 8.3. Clarke and Nicholson (2010) identified five key elements of resilience each of which is associated with distinctive attitudes and behaviours:

Table 8.4   Factors that promote or inhibit resilience.

Factors that promote resilience	Factors that inhibit resilience
Sense of humour	Humourless, hopeless, self-pity
Humility	Self-absorbed
Balanced	Extremist
Creative	Isolated
Autonomous	Dependent
Healthy relationships	Pattern of behaviour
Self-motivated	Passive
Content	Discontented/resigned

1. Optimism, a positive attitude and self-confidence
2. Freedom from stress and anxiety
3. Individual accountability
4. Openness and flexibility
5. Problem orientation.

Health professionals can enhance their personal resilience (Table 8.4) using these tools too, as well as through continued professional development.

Competencies and attributes health professionals need to manage their own transitions and help people with diabetes manage transitions
Health professionals need relevant knowledge about diabetes and education techniques (Chapters 1–3 and 10), understanding about psychological issues (Chapters 2 and 4), be self-actualised, aware of their own life stage and adaptation process, possess the relevant emotional and social intelligence and the capacity to communicate.

Social intelligence refers to social awareness and social facility (Goleman 2007). Social awareness encompasses the ability to:

- Sense another person's inner state
- Show empathy and understand the other person's feelings and reasons without becoming enmeshed
- Be present and connected to another person through active listening (Chapters 5 and 6)
- Know how society and health services function
- Understand the individual's support network and social coherence.

However, these abilities are not sufficient in themselves to develop a therapeutic relationship likely to help the individual cope with a transition (Chapter 5). Social facility is needed and builds on social awareness. Social facility includes:

- Communicating effectively using verbal and non-verbal language (Chapter 6), which Goleman (2007) referred to as synchrony.
- The ability to present themselves effectively.

- The capacity to influence the outcome of social interactions without being dictatorial or manipulative—*lead the individual to the threshold of their own mind* (Kahil Gibran 2008).
- Caring for other people's needs and using strategies to help them address their needs.

In the summary of a report of teacher round-table discussions (Snyder 2005), the Dean of the commissioning university highlighted two teacher's comments that resonated with him:

> *Ultimately, what he wanted teachers to know is that children do things for a reason and to understand that a teacher's job is to figure out those reasons and to use that knowledge to create contexts that support the growth and development of their students.*

The dean acknowledged 'that is a simply stated but difficult to do definition of one of the core functions of teacher education' (Snyder 2005, pp. v–vi).

The second teacher said:

> *Human beings are vulnerable and bring with them both risk and protective factors. The teacher's job is to create contexts that alleviate the risks and enrich the protective factors to support the growth and development of their students.*

These comments also apply to health professionals and people with diabetes. They highlight the need to create the conditions in which people with

---

Reflective questions

Reflection is essential to learning. It is a key part of the person with diabetes' journey and it is equally important for health professionals to reflect on their journey as carers and educators. The following statements or questions may help you reflect. It sometimes helps if you think about a recent encounter with a person with diabetes where you felt the encounter did not go as well as you would like.

- Do you think it is important to understand the ages and stages of life to develop individualised, holistic diabetes education and care?
- What reasons could you give to support your point of view?
- Think of a life transition you had. Was it positive or negative?
- What strategies did you use to manage the transition?
- Do you ever consider adult life transition stage when taking a health history and educating and caring for people with diabetes?
- How could you incorporate the arts into your practice to support people with diabetes to negotiate transitions?

diabetes can learn, including learning about who they are. If educators are to empower all individuals to learn, they must know and be able to apply information from human development and cognitive science within their own professional practice. Diabetes educator training curricula could include activities that involve reading and discussing books and movies that portray major life transitions such as those cited in this chapter and in Appendix.

Life is pleasant. Death is peaceful. It's the transition that's troublesome.

Isaac Asimov (1920–1992)

References

Antonovsky A. (1979) *Health, Stress and Coping*. San Francisco, CA: Jossey-Bass.

Antonovsky A. (1987) *Unraveling the Mystery of Health. How People Manage Stress and Stay Well*. San Francisco, CA: Jossey-Bass.

Bailey E. (2011) *The Sound of a Wild Snail Eating*. Melbourne: Text Publishing.

Bauby J-D. (1997) *The Diving Bell and The Butterfly*. New York: Knopf Doubleday.

Bridges W. (1991) *Transitions: Making Sense of Life's Changes*. Reading, MA: Addison Wesley.

Clarke J, Nicholson J. (2010) *Resilience: Bounce Back from Whatever Life Throws at You*. Kuala Lumpur: Advantage Quest Publications.

Dilts R. (1990) *Changing Belief Systems with NLP*. Capitola, CA: Meta Publications.

Dunning T. (2009) *Car of People with Diabetes: A Manual of Nursing Practice*. Chichester, Wiley-Blackwell, pp. 39 and 420.

Eliot T. (1950) *The Cocktail Party: A Comedy*. London: Faber and Faber.

Emotional Wellness Matters. (1999–2004) Life transitions. http://lifeesteem. org/wellness/wellnessLF.html (accessed January 2012).

Eos Career Services LifeLine Chart. (1997–2001) http://www.eoslifework. co.uk/transmgmt1.html (accessed February 2012).

Epictetus. (unknown) *Springs of Greek Wisdom*. New York: Herder and Herder.

Erikson E. (1950) *Childhood and Society*. New York: Norton Books.

Frankl V. (1969) *The Will to Meaning: Foundations and Applications of Logotherapy*. London: Meridian.

Gibran K. (2008) *Kahlil Gibran's the Prophet and the Art of Peace*. The new illustrated edition. London: Duncan Baird Publishers, p. 99.

Goleman D. (2007) *Social Intelligence*. London: Random House.

Homer. (1966) *Springs of Greek Wisdom*. New York: Herder and Herder.

Khayyam O. (1965) *The Rubaiyat of Omar Khayyam*, Translated by Edward Fitzgerald. London: Ward, Lock & Co Limited.

Kubler-Ross E. (1969) *On Death and Dying*. London: Routledge.

Levine P. (2008) *Cycle of Life: Creating Smooth Passages in Everyday Life*. Ukiah, CA: The Nourishing Company.

Levinson D. (1978) *Seasons of a Man's Life*. New York: Knopf.

Mair V. (2009) Pinyin information danger + opportunity = crisis: Has misunderstanding of Chinese characters led many astray? http://pinyin.infolinks. html (accessed January 2012).

Marina-Tompkins V. (2011) *Spiritual Turning Points: A Metaphysical Perspective of the Seven Life Transitions*. Victoria: Marina-Tompkins Xlibris.

Rasmussen B, O'Connell B, Dunning T. (2007) Young women with type 1 diabetes' management of turning points and transition. *Qualitative Health Research* 17(3):300–310.

Rogers C. (1991) *On Becoming a Person: A Therapists View of Psychotherapy*. Boston, MA: Houghton Mifflin.

Sacks O. (1985) *The Man Who Mistook His Wife for a Hat: And Other Clinical Tales*. London: Pan MacMillan.

Seuss. (1990) *On the Places You Go*. New York: Random House.

Shakespeare W. (1964) As you like it. In *The Complete Works of William Shakespeare*, The Players Edition, Alexander P. (ed.). London and Edinburgh: Collins.

Sheehy G. (1995) *Passages: Predictable Crises of Adult Life*. New York: Bantam.

Skinner B. (1971) *Beyond Freedom and Dignity*. Indianapolis, IN: Hackett.

Snyder J. (2005) Dean's comment in Child and adolescent developmental research of teacher education: Evidence-based pedagogy, policy and practice. Summary of roundtable discussion 2005 and 2006. Rockville, MD: National Institute of Child Health and Human Development and National Council for Teacher Education, pp. v–vi.

Spinoza. (1970) *Spirit of Sagittarius*. New York: Herder and Herder.

Stout G. (2009) The living years. www.theliving yearsjournal.com (accessed November 2011).

Sugarman L. (2004) *Counselling and the Life Course*. London: Sage.

Williams D. (January 1999) Life events and career change: Transition psychology in practice. Presentation at the British Psychological Society, London.

9 Sharing Stories of the Journey: Peer Education

Gretchen A. Piatt[1,2], Rhonda Lee[3], Helen Thomasic[3],
Norma Ryan[3] and Millie Glinsky[4]

[1] Division of Endocrinology and Metabolism, School of Medicine, University of
Pittsburgh, Pittsburgh, PA, USA
[2] Diabetes Institute, University of Pittsburgh, Pittsburgh, PA, USA
[3] Medical Center, University of Pittsburgh, Pittsburgh, PA, USA
[4] Indiana Regional Medical Center, Indiana, PA, USA

> *In all people I see myself—none more, and not one a barleycorn less;*
> *And the good or bad I say of myself, I say of them …*
>
> Walt Whitman (1891)

Introduction

Diabetes is a serious disease that requires a person to make daily decisions
about their self-care and that includes behaviours such as nutrition, exercise, risk reduction, coping, monitoring, problem-solving and medication
adherence. A body of evidence demonstrates that interventions that foster
diabetes self-management improve health status and lower healthcare
costs (Brown et al. 1999).

Diabetes self-management education (DSME) is critical in laying the
foundation for promoting the knowledge and skills for patients to perform
self-care tasks. DSME improves outcomes (Brown et al. 1999; Norris et al.
2002) and the effectiveness of DSME is directly associated with the amount
of time spent with the diabetes educator. Although improvements in
HbA_{1c} values are observed following DSME, benefits tend to decrease
1–3 months later (Norris et al. 2002). This suggests that DSME alone may
not be sufficient to maintain improved behaviours over a lifetime and sustained improvement requires time, contact and follow-up.

DSME is now more patient-centred and theoretically based; therefore
programmes are now putting greater emphasis on providing ongoing support to sustain DSME gains (Siminerio et al. 2006a; Funnell 2010) and

Diabetes Education: Art, Science and Evidence, First Edition. Edited by Trisha Dunning AM.
© 2013 John Wiley & Sons, Ltd. Published 2013 by John Wiley & Sons, Ltd.

attempting to incorporate self-management support (SMS) into their structure (Glasgow 1995; Wagner 2000; Anderson 2005). Despite efforts and evidence that DSME is important and attempts for sustained follow-up are being made, the numbers of DSME programmes and educators to provide these services are shrinking while the rates of diabetes are increasing (Anderson 1994; Conrood et al. 1994; Hiss et al. 1994; Mensing et al. 2006). Thus, opportunities for comprehensive services that increase access and include SMS are critical.

There is a growing body of literature that provides evidence for the utilisation of peer leaders as part of the diabetes care delivery system (Heisler et al. 2005; Tang et al. 2005). Peer leaders are used effectively to assist in self-management, provide social and emotional support and cultural mediation, link people to the health system, and provide ongoing support to help people management their disease (Lorig et al. 1999; Tang et al. 2005). The use of peer leaders provides a potentially low-cost, flexible means to supplement health care. If carefully designed and implemented, peer leader initiatives can be a powerful way to help patients with diabetes live more successfully.

In the face of growing numbers of people with diabetes and significant resource constraints facing health systems worldwide, it is increasingly important to develop and evaluate low-cost initiatives that build on available resources. Peer leaders provide a unique opportunity to serve as a resource for ongoing community-based self-management support initiatives; however, many questions regarding their role in a model of diabetes care delivery remain unanswered. These include questions surrounding the advantages and disadvantages of using peer leaders in ongoing diabetes delivery systems and the need to support and nurture the peer leader. Moreover, it is critical to explore the role of empathy and its influences on clinical and behaviour change, and whether diabetes educators who have diabetes themselves should indeed be considered peer leaders.

The use of peer leaders in diabetes self-management

As health systems around the world strive to transition from systems that focus on acute care management to chronic illness prevention and health promotion, a subset of individuals (peer leaders) are emerging as a potential solution to help to improve diabetes care and quality of life. Merriam-Webster defines the term 'peer' as 'one that is of equal standing with another; especially: one belonging to the same societal group especially based on age, grade, or status'. Tangential to the term 'peer', the term 'support' is defined by Merriam-Webster as 'one that supports—often used attributively'.

Therefore, peer support may be defined as the giving of support or assistance by one who is considered equal. More formally, Dennis (2002) developed a comprehensive definition of peer support in the healthcare context. According to this definition, peer support is '… the provision of emotional, appraisal and informational assistance by a created social network member who possesses experiential knowledge of a specific behavior or stressor and similar characteristics as the target population'.

Peer leaders, sometimes referred to as community health workers, lay health coaches, *promatores de salud*, etc., are individuals who share common characteristics with a 'targeted' group or individual, allowing them to relate to and empathise with that individual on a level that a non-peer would not be able to (Doull et al. 2007). Common characteristics of peer leaders include age, gender, disease status, socioeconomic status, religion, ethnicity, place of residence, and culture or education.

Peer leaders often demonstrate that they carry wisdom and experience about their chronic diseases, including diabetes that far exceeds their physicians and other healthcare providers too (Doull et al. 2007). They are oftentimes patients who are able to successfully deal with the problems posed by their diabetes and who maintain a positive lifestyle. Peer leaders often share common traits such as the ability to develop relationships, sufficient time availability, along with being empathetic and motivated (Boothroyd and Fisher 2010 a,b). These individuals may live longer, are healthier and are a great resource and source of support to other individuals with diabetes (Donaldson 2003).

Due to limited financial resources in healthcare systems and the worldwide pandemic of diabetes, peer support is becoming an increasingly important strategy to provide low-cost scalable interventions aimed at promoting self-management support to improve diabetes care and outcomes. With estimates of 300–350 million people with diabetes, worldwide, by 2025 (Clark 2010), it is no longer feasible to continue to increase the number physicians, nurses, dietitians and healthcare facilities to attempt to curtail the rising incidence and prevalence of the disease. As such, the World Health Organization (WHO) acknowledged social support as a critical component of health promotion and recently, 2008, formed a consultation on peer support programmes in diabetes. The WHO (2007) now recognises peer support as an effective approach to diabetes management.

Individuals with diabetes manage nearly 99% of their disease on their own (Anderson et al.1994; Funnell and Anderson 2003; Funnell 2010), with the patients and their families baring the responsibility for daily self-management. A number of behaviours that patients need to successfully execute, on a daily basis, in order to successfully self-manage their diabetes—taking prescribed medications, following diet and exercise regimens, self-monitoring blood glucose and coping emotionally with the challenges of having diabetes. Many patients with diabetes have a difficult time carrying out these behaviours, and moreover, they may lack adequate support from family and friends to help them with their diabetes self-management (Piatt et al. 2006; Heisler 2010).

Evidence demonstrates that diabetes education and self-management (DSME) have a positive impact on patients' clinical, behavioural and psychosocial outcomes (Siminerio et al. 2005; Siminerio 2006 a,b; Piatt et al. 2006) and that DSME is a cost-effective adjunct to medical care (American Association of Diabetes Educators (AADE) 2010). However, with the pandemic of diabetes and the ever-growing incidence of the disease, it is increasingly more difficult for diabetes educators to meet the high demand. Additionally, attending DSME is often times not 'enough' for positive behaviour change to be sustained (Funnell 2010).

Often, there are a number of barriers that patients face to attending traditional face-to-face group or individual DSME sessions. Most notably, DSME sessions are time-limited, often leading to increase lack of attendance and long-term support (Heisler 2007, 2010; Heisler et al. 2010). Thus, the integration of peer leaders into the diabetes self-management network can effectively reach more people with diabetes and provide ongoing self-management support. Additionally, evidence suggests that higher levels of social support, which are illness or regimen-specific, are associated with improved diabetes self-management (Glasgow and Toobert 1988; Ruggiero et al. 1990; Tillotson and Smith 1996).

Several studies have demonstrated that peer support contributes to improvements in medication adherence, diet, exercise and blood glucose monitoring (Wilson et al. 1986; Joseph et al. 2001; Samuel-Hodge et al. 2000; Peers for Progress 2010). If integrated with appropriate planning, oversight and training, the use of peer leaders may lead to sustained behaviour change and a sustainable model of DSME.

The most effective peer support models appear to combine peer support with a structured programme of DSME (Heisler 2010; Heisler et al. 2010) and are delivered through multiple modes of interaction, including modes such as individual and group sessions, self-help/support groups and Internet groups. The programmes are often implemented in diverse settings, such as the home, community organisation, school, or via telephone or internet and the role of the peer leader may take the form of an educator, coach or liaison (Dennis 2002). Although there are several modalities of how and where to implement peer support, actual provision of peer support comprises four main attributes that are applicable to all settings and modes of delivery.

There is no 'one size fits all' approach to implementing peer support because of the vast array of cultural and demographic differences of peer leaders; however, the following four functions, developed by the Peers for Progress (Boothroyd and Fisher 2010a; Peers for Progress 2010) initiative, offer a standardised structure in which peer support programmes may be built and evaluated. Within the scope of DSME, the four key functions of a peer leader are to

1. Assist in self-management
2. Provide social and emotional support

3. Link patients to clinical care
4. Provide ongoing support (Boothroyd and Fisher 2010a; Peers for Progress 2010).

When a peer leader assists in self-management, they help patients to apply and incorporate the concepts of DSME into their daily lives (Fisher et al. 2005). This is achieved by using a number of educational and psychological tools including goal setting, skill building, practising and rehearsal of behaviours, trouble-shooting barriers and challenges, and problem solving. Peer leaders also often work on practising healthy eating habits and being physically active with the patients so that there is a reciprocal support mechanism.

A critical function of a peer leader is also to provide social and emotional support (Boothroyd and Fisher 2010 a,b). Strong evidence exists that there is a direct association between increased social support and improved health outcomes. In fact, social support is often considered a protective factor in health and may be as important as negative factors, e.g. obesity, smoking and hypertension (Boothroyd and Fisher 2010 a,b). When providing social and emotional support, peer leaders maintain frequent contact with patients, encourage patients to use their self-management skills and also how to effectively deal with diabetes and non-diabetes-related stress. Above all else, peer leaders are simply available to talk with people troubled by negative emotions.

This aspect is especially critical for patients who may lack an extensive social network (e.g. family and friends) to provide diabetes support or for patients with a social network that is not supportive of their self-management efforts. The elderly especially fall victim to not having a social network, and often as a consequence, they experience higher rates of depression than the general population (Malchodi et al. 2003; Heisler 2010).

The third key function of peer support is for the peer leader to act as a liaison or link to clinical care (Booothroyd and Fisher 2010 a,b). This function of peer support can be divided into two over-arching categories: (1) the linkages the peer leader develops and maintains in the primary care practice setting or other clinical care settings and (2) encouragement for patients to receive regular clinical care and form partnerships with their clinical care providers.

As the majority of diabetes care is delivered within the primary care practice setting, establishing relationships in this setting is critical. For example, the peer leader may often serve dual roles by reminding providers and office staff.about the standard clinical care guidelines, and by also reminding patients of regularly scheduled appointments, encouraging timely provider visits and ensuring that patients are aware of the recommended testing that should be provided for people with diabetes.

The final function of a peer leader is to provide ongoing support (Boothroyd and Fisher 2010 a,b). Research demonstrates that DSME is effective in improving patient self-care behaviours and clinical outcomes, including H6A1c. However, these effects often diminish within 1–3 months after DSME ends (Siminerio et al. 2006b; Norris et al. 2006). Proactive, ongoing support is critical for patients to maintain improvements and work on sustaining lifestyle modifications. Peer leaders offer a flexible, non-threatening, low-cost alternative to traditional follow-up strategies. Patients are encouraged to utilise their peer leader on an as-needed basis for as long as they need, to help and support their self-care goals.

Two peer leaders wrote the following passage. It provides insight into how peer leaders feel about their role in helping to improve diabetes care. Similar passages appear throughout this chapter.

Story of the Journey (Rhonda Lee and Helen Thomasic, Lifestyle Coaches, Pittsburgh, Pennsylvania)

The textbook definition cannot fully describe what it means to be a peer leader or lifestyle coach. We are more than coaches; we are advocates, cheerleaders, and friends. Our job is to motivate and inspire people to make positive changes in their lives. As part of our job, we provide support and practical information as well as relevant personal experiences about making behavior changes. Making a behavior change is difficult and our program participants need a lot of guidance and encouragement. When you have been living your life a certain way for years it can be hard to make changes to the way you think, eat, and exercise.

First and foremost, we want you to know that you are not alone. Our mission is to encourage, support and listen as well as provide answers to your questions. As lifestyle coaches, we are there to hold your hand, to lend an ear and to guide your diabetes self-management. But, it doesn't end there. As your coach, we are only a phone call away. When you feel you have come upon a slippery slope, we are here to help and encourage you to start again. We will help you take what you have learned during the classes and incorporate it into your daily life. We try to be open-minded and to really get to know you so we can understand the obstacles that you need to overcome. Our hope is that a cure for diabetes will be found in our lifetime. However, until that day comes, we will continue to focus our efforts on helping people to make positive behavior changes. As lifestyle coaches, we have the knowledge to help people change their lives and for us that is the most rewarding job of all.

Supporting and educating the peer leader

It is crucial for peer leaders to receive standardised training in order for them to build the skills and competencies for delivering self-management support. Most people with one or multiple chronic illnesses have problems self-managing their disease at one time or another throughout their lifetime; however, usually, they find a way to cope with these problems. It is during these problem times, though, that the use of peer leaders is particularly crucial. With standardised training and support from healthcare professionals, peer leaders offer a vehicle to enable patients to reduce their levels of stress through emotional support, access appropriate and accessible education material and clinical care, and receive required services that allows the mobilisation of multiple resources, and ultimately improved self-care.

The concept of using peer leaders for self-management support is not a new one. Peer leaders have been used across multiple disease states to provide support for HIV/AIDS patients, drug abuse prevention, tobacco cessation and on university campuses worldwide, to name a few (Swider 2002; Norris et al. 2006). However, it was only in the past decade that peer leaders gained attention in the field of DSME. In the United States, there are approximately 15,000 certified diabetes educators (CDEs) to serve the 25.8 million people with diabetes (AADE 2010).

That means there is approximately one CDE for every 1720 patients with diabetes—a daunting ratio for any healthcare professional. This disparate ratio exemplifies the necessity for healthcare systems to embrace low cost, flexible ways of dealing with the diabetes epidemic. The use of peer leaders to supplement the role of the CDE provides an opportunity to increase access to diabetes self-management support services and serves as a vehicle to defragment the part of the healthcare system that focuses on self-management support health services delivery (Conrood et al. 1994; Hiss et al. 1994; Mensing et al. 2006).

With the growing diabetes epidemic, healthcare professionals, communities and health systems, worldwide, began utilising peer leaders in their diabetes programmes, research studies and daily operations. However, for the most part, the focus remained on implementing these efforts rather than the training and education processes that are necessary for individuals to serve as peer leaders (Tang et al. 2011). Of the studies that report a standardised training component to their programme or intervention, few provide a description of the process (Joshu et al. 2007; Paul et al. 2007 a,b; Brownson and Heisler 2009: Dale et al. 2009; Tang et al. 2011). An exception to this is Project Dulce (Philis-Tsimikas et al. 2004) and the Stanford Diabetes Self Management Program (DSMP) (Lorig et al. 1999; Holman and Lorig 2000 a,b) that utilise a standardised curriculum, are evidence-based and are measurable. Both initiatives focus on training peer leaders to deliver short duration DSME programmes; however, what they lack is a focus on providing long-term self-management support (Tang et al. 2011), a concept that has been proven to be one of the cornerstones of effective diabetes care (Piatt et al. 2010).

Additionally, efforts aimed at standardising these initiatives so that they are measurable and can be replicated across settings and populations remains sparse. Nettles and Belton (2010), in their review of training curricula for diabetes peer educators, found that all peer education programmes provided training in some capacity; however, the details of the training (i.e. length, evaluation, fidelity) varied widely and few programmes conducted formal evaluation plans.

While characteristics of the training vary, there is consensus from the literature that peer leaders need to be able to communicate effectively, be willing to learn, have confidence in diabetes content and be flexible and dependable (Nettles and Belton 2010) in order to deliver effective peer education. While many of these characteristics are innate, standardised curriculum and training complement these factors, helping to ensure long-term self-management support and sustainability.

In developing a peer-training curriculum, it is important to first understand and determine the role of the peer leader. Depending on whether the peer leader will educate, facilitate or counsel will determine the type of training they should receive (Peers for Progress 2010). In general, one way for peer leaders to understand their designated role in self-management support is by practising active listening through the OARS:

- Ask **O**pen-ended questions
- **A**ffirm
- **R**eflect
- **S**ummarise.

Is a motivational interviewing strategy often used in communicating with individuals who are trying to make a behaviour change (Miller 2009)? Tangential to OARS, peer leaders may also set SMART goals for themselves to better understand their role in self-management support (Tang et al. 2011):

- **S**pecific
- **M**easurable
- **A**chievable
- **R**ealistic
- **T**ake the right amount of time (see Chapter 4).

Common concepts that are addressed in a thorough peer leader training curriculum include understanding of problem solving skills, communication skills, decision-making skills, finding healthcare resources, developing goal plans for the future, understanding the management principles of diabetes self-care, and understanding and managing psychosocial responses to diabetes (Tang et al. 2011). Through training, peer leaders will acquire supportive skills to help them to assist patients who are experiencing a variety of circumstances in their diabetes self-management. They will learn new and different ways to communicate and new techniques for dealing with emotionally charged issues.

Through active listening and setting SMART goals, peer leaders will be able to understand how patients are coping with their emotions and how to help them cope in times of particular diabetes-related distress. A standardised training curriculum also affords the peer leaders with the opportunity to learn by practice, in group sessions, when a situation requires professional intervention, a concept that is critical in peer support interventions and programmes. Training allows peer leaders to recognise when a crisis is a crisis (i.e. hypoglycaemic or major depressive episodes, or a patient who may have thoughts of suicide), and what resources are available in the community for these issues.

Along with understanding the patient, individuals who assume the role of a peer leader have certain responsibilities to themselves, the programme and the agency (Peers for Progress 2010). It is critical that these concepts are covered in the training curriculum. First and foremost, peer leaders need to be able to acknowledge their limitations. These limitations and challenges could include time commitments, the balance between training burden and volunteer status, monetary incentive amounts and literacy. Additionally, as most peer leader programmes are 'housed' within a research study, it is important for peer leaders to understand and be competent in human subject research interactions. Handling patient information and understanding privacy and confidentiality are components that are crucial in this setting (Halanych and Moultry 2010). If these concepts are taken into consideration during the training, the peer leaders will be apprised of their importance before the start of the programme.

In summary, training for peer support should pay attention to the aforementioned framework and address core competencies and functions of peer support as outlined in the World Health Organization's report on peer support programmes in diabetes. These peer leader core competencies include assistance in diabetes management in daily living, social and emotional support, linkages to care and ongoing support extended over time. While these competencies apply to any peer support programme, specific approaches to addressing them may vary based on the needs and contexts of different populations and settings.

Story of the Journey (Norma Ryan, Lay Health Coach, Brownsville, Pennsylvania)

When I first heard the words of 'Lay Health Coach' I shuttered to wonder what that could mean. After a year of spending time with study participants, I am quite sure that the role of a lay health coach plays a very important part in diabetes management. My belief is that lay health coaches are people in the community who are known as a 'friend' and patients are often more comfortable sharing the good and bad of their concerns with them.

Often people feel a little intimidated to talk to a professional doctor or nurse, but that friend on the street is someone like them and they are more apt to share their failures and quick to share successes. This experience of being a lay health coach has been a very rewarding time in my life. I have learned so much that I am now able to share with family and friends. I want you to know that I am so very thrilled to have been part of this and would love to continue to help others live a healthy lifestyle. This is the beginning of a new 'era' of me sharing experience and knowledge with family and friends.

I *am* You: Understanding empathy in the field of peer education

Hojat (2007) defines empathy as 'the projection of feelings that turn I **and** you into I **am** you, or at least I **might** be you'. Empathy grows throughout one's lifetime and is more than a neurobiological response. Indeed, it brings feelings with it and helps individuals to understand who they are (Hojat 2007). The term empathy has gone through many deviations, often being thought of as a cognitive attribute, which allows individuals to understand each other, or as an emotional state of mind where individuals are more likely to share feelings, or as a concept that involves both cognition and emotion. Regardless of the definition, empathy is among the most frequently mentioned dimensions of patient care (Linn et al. 1987; Hojat 2007) and is quite possibly, the single most important component of a successful peer leader.

Empathy and sympathy

In understanding the role of empathy in peer education, it is important to distinguish between sympathy and empathy, a concept that is often confused. While both sympathy and empathy are emotional responses, empathy carries with it a clear separation between emotion and cognition. When effective peer leaders interact with patients, they are able to non-judgmentally understand the patients' experiences and recognise that they is similar to them (i.e. they have diabetes, live in the same community, same age range, etc.), while maintaining a clear separation. This separation is what distinguishes empathy from sympathy, as empathy is an intellectual attribute and sympathy is an emotional state of mind (Gruen and Mendelsohn 1986; Hojat 2007). Empathetic peer leaders are able to separate themselves from the patients' self-management issues and offer information and advice to improve self-care; whereas, sympathetic peer leaders have difficulty in maintaining whose feelings belong to whom (Decety and Jackson 2004; Hojat 2007).

Empathy and social support

Social support is defined as a multidimensional construct of social relationships that enhances well-being (Rodriguez and Cohen 1998) and can be thought of as the relationships that individuals have within and among family, friends, the workplace, the community and the health system. Morgan (Morgan 2002) believes that a strong, functional support system requires empathy at its core (Hojat 2007). Central to this belief is that a social support system provides cognitive and emotional resources that benefit an individual's ability to cope with stress (Rodriguez and Cohen 1998). In fact, there is significant evidence that demonstrates that social support is either directly or indirectly related to improved physical, mental and social well-being, the three cornerstone elements of the World Health

Organization's definition of 'health'. Likewise, research demonstrates the risk of physical illness worsening, when a person's social connection becomes weak or fragmented (Hojat 2007).

When we think about how peer leaders function among patients with diabetes, it is clear that they provide an outlet for people to talk about the concerns and feelings they have about their self-management. This relationship is often formed by the need for personal connection that increases with illness. The empathic connection between a patient and a peer leader may serve as an independent social support system (Hojat 2007). Patients are able to 'open-up' to peer leaders, because in general peer leaders possess high degrees of active listening skills and work on maintaining empathetic connections with the patients. It is through this empathetic connection within a positive, social support system, that patients often begin to reflect on their barriers and challenges to diabetes self-management at deeper levels, which in turn may lead to a positive health outcome.

Empathy and patient relationships

It is well documented in the medical literature that clinicians as well as patients may benefit from empathic engagement (Hojat 2007). So, it stands to reason that the same scenario may be present for peer leaders. During times of understanding and connectedness between the patient and the peer leader, physiological and emotional responses may be apparent. Patients may feel that they are immediately 'understood', as if the peer leader is experiencing the situation from inside the patient's world, by a sense of being part of a larger whole and by feelings of peacefulness that relate to connecting to someone who truly understands them. These moments may be therapeutic for both the patient and the peer leader and may lead to improved diabetes self-care for both individuals.

Evolution has taught human beings to be social and it is through evolution that humans have the ability to understand others and the skills to communicate that understanding (Hojat 2007). The connections that humans have with each other are the cornerstone for empathetic growth.

Story of the Journey (Millie Glinsky, Lay Health Coach, Indiana, Pennsylvania)

When developing my most recent coaching 'curriculum' for a series of sessions I am currently conducting, I titled it 'Value Yourself—one small change changes everything'. I was excited about the series because the sequence was planned to build a focus on making lifestyle changes in the 'big 3' areas. The 'big 3' of course being exercise, nutrition and stress management. Instead of developing exercise and calorie goals to lose weight and get healthy, I asked patients to write down what it means to 'value yourself' and these responses would be compared to responses to the same question at the end of the ten week series.

What I was not prepared for was the intimate and trusting class environment that happened early in the program. Men and women who didn't know one another in the first class were sharing personal fears and disappointments by the third meeting. Each personal weekly goal was met with a feeling of group support and encouragement. Successes were applauded and struggles were examined for possible redirection and solutions. Although I acted as guide and leader, discussions and insights came from the patients. In working through many of their shared concerns and previous 'failures' at losing weight, everyone developed a more tolerant attitude toward themselves that paved the way for improved lifestyle choices and behavior change.

As predicted, the responses to the original question of what it means to 'value yourself' changed dramatically by the end of the ten week series. Patients learned about themselves, about one another and also about me, as their coach. But the greatest surprise of all was how much I learned from them, which, for me, holds the greatest value in helping others become more who they are meant to be.

I'm a diabetes educator who has diabetes—can I be a peer leader?

Peer leaders are individuals who have knowledge from their own experience with diabetes or from family members or close friends who may have the disease. In most circumstances, peer leaders have experienced success in their own diabetes self-management or have helped others to experience success. Although many healthcare systems, worldwide, are recognising peer leaders as critical components of the healthcare team, the main function of a peer leader is to provide support, not to make healthcare recommendations that only professionals, such as diabetes educators, could make (Lorig et al. 1999; Holman and Lorig 2000 a,b; AADE 2010). Peer leaders serve as a 'complement' to clinical care and diabetes self-management education, not as a replacement.

It is well documented in the literature that DSME is effective and leads to both clinical and behavioural improvements in diabetes self-management (Norris et al. 2002; Siminerio et al. 2005; Siminerio et al. 2006 a,b; Piatt et al. 2006, 2010). However, scientific evidence is beginning to accumulate that demonstrates additional benefit from learning from peer leaders—individuals who are living the experience everyday and are facing the same issues in navigating the health system, handling finances and dealing with emotions and family dynamics (Boothroyd and Fisher 2010 a,b; Peers for Progress 2010).

Norris et al. (2006) documented in her 2006 review of 18 studies using peer leaders that participants were satisfied with their peer leader and their diabetes knowledge improved. Additionally, improvements in physiologic, lifestyle and self-care outcomes were noted. These improvements, however, do not discount the effectiveness or impact of the diabetes educator.

As the epidemic of diabetes continues to worsen, diabetes educators may effectively reach more people with diabetes by expanding their education team to include peer leaders, not serving in the peer leader role themselves (AADE 2010). As the peer leader evidence demonstrates, having diabetes is not enough to qualify someone as a peer leader. Peer leaders live, work and function in the communities in which their patients live. Self-management support delivered by peer leaders often takes place in community settings, such as churches, community centres, fire halls and schools, which are convenient and familiar to patients (Holman and Lorig 2000a,b). Additionally, unlike diabetes education, peer leader self-management support often takes place during off hours or on weekends, or even by phone or email and is by and far not clinical in nature.

Indeed, peer leaders mostly work on goal setting and problem solving with patients, not providing clinical advice. And most importantly, peer leaders are people who are known in the community, trusted and culturally competent. They understand the barriers and challenges that people with diabetes face in their respective communities and are able to offer alternatives and suggestions to help patients in dealing with their diabetes. Peer leaders are usually never health professionals. Indeed, they are often retirees or homemakers with a special interest in diabetes and are personable, empathetic and communicate well (Philis-Tsimikas et al. 2004; Halanych and Moultry 2010; Peers for Progress 2010).

In contrast, diabetes educators who have diabetes have years of experience working within a healthcare system and have a deep knowledge and understanding of diabetes. Therefore, they may not be able to convey the sense of support and camaraderie that patients need. Indeed, it is often the case that patients will seek out the peer leader to ask a question, rather than the diabetes educator for fear that the educator may judge them or give them information that does not pertain to their situation.

Scientific and programmatic evidence continues to build for the incorporation and utilisation of peer leaders within the healthcare system. Not only do they provide a low-cost, flexible means of increasing access to diabetes-related services, but they also provide an opportunity for long-term diabetes self-management support, which is currently not being addressed. The American Association of Diabetes Educators suggests that in order to meet the demands of the diabetes epidemic, diabetes educators and CDEs, regardless of their diabetes status, should incorporate peer leaders into their diabetes education team to help to curtail the ever-worsening diabetes epidemic.

The following passages were written by patients who are part of a research study focused on testing the effectiveness of peer leaders within a diabetes care delivery system (Piatt et al. 2010). They underscore the main differences between peer leaders and diabetes educators, from a patient perspective.

Story of the Journey (Study Participant, Project SEED: Support, Education, and Evaluation in Diabetes)

I think of my peer leader as a friend; as someone we can relate to cause of her diabetes. She tries to relate to each of us in the study group. When we talk on the phone, which is very helpful, she always tries to bolster your spirits. She also shares her own ups and downs. Always ready with ways she can help you.

I feel that my diabetes educator is the professional—someone who I can trust with my diabetes and issues. She is like having my own doctor at the meetings. She always answers everyone's questions with a certain layperson appeal. She breaks down answers to our questions so we can understand our diabetes. My diabetes educator has personally helped me better understand my diabetes.

Both my peer leader and my diabetes educator are an asset to our group.

Story of the Journey (Study Participant, Project SEED: Support, Education, and Evaluation in Diabetes)

My peer leader has knowledge through experience of diabetes. My diabetes educator's knowledge comes from educational learning and training.

My peer leader's obvious compassion for others with this affliction and her willingness to help is a blessing.

Reflective questions

Reflection is essential to learning. It is a key part of the person with diabetes' journey and it is equally important for health professionals to reflect on their journey as carers and educators. The following statements or questions may help you reflect. It sometimes helps if you think about a recent encounter with a person with diabetes where you felt the encounter did not go as well as you would like.

- DSME is now more patient-centred and theoretically based; therefore, programmes are putting greater emphasis on providing ongoing support to sustain DSME gains and attempting to incorporate self-management support into their structure. What is your diabetes centre doing to help to incorporate ongoing self-management support?
- Peer leaders are individuals who share common characteristics with a targeted group or individual, allowing them to relate to and empathise with that individual on a level that a non-peer would not be able to. Reflect on your patients and their personalities. Who do you think would fit the role of a peer leader?
- In reflecting on your role, as an educator, think about the differences between you and a potential peer leader and reflect on the physical and emotional resources that a peer leader may be able to provide for your patients, that you, as an educator, may not have time to provide.
- How do you think addition of the peer leader to the healthcare team may lead to long-term sustainability of self-management support?

References

American Association of Diabetes Educators. (2010) A sustainable model of diabetes self-management education/training involves a multi-level team that can include community health workers, Chicago, IL.

Anderson, C. (1994) Measuring what works in health care, *Science* 263: 1080–1082.

Anderson, R.M. (2005) Is it ethical to assign medically underserved African Americans to a usual-care control group in community-based intervention research? *Diabetes Care* 28(7): 1817–1820.

Anderson, R.M., Hiss, R.G., Stephen, C.J., Fitzgerald, J.T., and Funnell, M.M. (1994) The diabetes education experience of randomly selected patients under the care of community physicians, *The Diabetes Educator* 20(5): 39–405.

Boothroyd, R. and Fisher, E.B. (2010a) Peers for progress: Promoting peer support for health around the world, *Family Practice*, 27(Suppl 1): i62–i68.

Boothroyd, R. and Fisher, E.B. (2010b) Generalizable functions of peer support & local tailoring of peer support interventions: Examples from peers for progress, in *Peer Support Across Cultural, National, & Organizational Settings: Common Functions and Setting-Specific Features*, International Society of Behavioral Medicine, Washington, DC.

Brown, J.B., Nichols, G.A., Glauber, H.S., and Bakst, A.W. (1999) Type 2 diabetes: Incremental medical care costs during the first 8 years after diagnosis, *Diabetes Care* 22(7): 1116–1124.

Brownson, C.A. and Heisler, M. (2009) The role of peer support in diabetes care and self management, *Patient Education and Counseling* 2: 5–17.

Clark, C.M. (2010) Overview, *Family Practice* 27(Suppl 1): i3–i5.

Conrood, B.A., Betschart, J., and Harris, M.I. (1994) Frequency and determinants of diabetes patient education among adults in the U.S. population, *Diabetes Care* 17(8): 822–858.

Dale, J., Caramalau, I., Sturt, J., Friede, T., Walker, R. (2009) Telephone peer-delivered intervention for diabetes motivation and support: The telecare exploratory RCT, *Patient Education and Counseling* 75: 91–98.

Decety, J. and Jackson, P.L. (2004) The functional architecture of human empathy, *Behavior and Cognitive Neuroscience Review* 3: 71–100.

Dennis, C. (2002) Peer support within a health care context: A concept analysis, *International Journal of Nursing Studies* 40: 321–332.

Donaldson, L. (2003) Expert patients usher in a new era of opportunity for the NHS, *British Medical Journal* 326: 1279.

Doull, M., O'Connor, A.M., Robinson, V., Tugwell, P., and Wells, G.A. (2007) Peer support strategies for improving health and well-being of individuals with chronic diseases, *Cochrane Database of Systematic Reviews* 3: CD005352.

Fisher, E.B., Brownson, C.A., O'Toole, M.L., Shetty, G., Anwuri, V.V., and Glasgow, R.E. (2005) Ecological approaches to self-management: The case of diabetes, *American Journal of Public Health* 95(9): 1523–1535.

Funnell, M.M. (2010) Peer-based behavioural strategies to improve chronic disease self-management and clinical outcomes: Evidence, logistics, evaluation considerations and needs for future research, *Family Practice* 27(suppl 1): i17–i22.

Funnell, M.M. and Anderson, R.M. (2003) Patient empowerment: A look back, a look ahead, *Diabetes Educator* 29(3): 454–460.

Glasgow, R.E. (1995) A practical model of diabetes management and education, *Diabetes Care* 18(1): 117–126.

Glasgow, R. and Toobert, D.J. (1988) Social environment and regimen adherence among type 2 diabetic patients, *Diabetes Care* 11: 377–386.

Gruen, R.J. and Mendelsohn, G. (1986) Emotional responses to affective displays in others: The distinction between empathy and sympathy, *Journal of Personality and Social Psychology* 51: 609–614.

Halanych, J. and Moultry, S. (2010) Encourage: Evaluating community peer advisors and diabetes outcomes in rural alabama, in *National Rural Health Association Conference*, Savannah, GA.

Heisler, M. (2007) Overview of peer support models to improve diabetes self-management and clinical outcomes, *Diabetes Spectrum* 20(4): 214–221.

Heisler, M. (2010) Different models to mobilize peer support to improve diabetes self-management and clinical outcomes: Evidence, logistics, evaluation considerations and needs for future research, *Family Practice* 27(suppl 1): i23–i32.

Heisler, M., Piette, J.D., Spencer, M., Kieffer, E., and Vijan, S. (2005) The relationship between knowledge of recent HbA1c values and diabetes care understanding and self-management, *Diabetes Care* 28(4): 816–822.

Heisler, M., Vijan, S., Makki, F., Piette, J. (2010) Diabetes control with reciprocal peer support versus nurse care management, *Annals of Internal Medicine* 153(8): 507–515.

Hiss, R.G. et al. (1994) Community diabetes care. A 10-year perspective, *Diabetes Care* 17(10): 1124–1133.

Hojat, M. (2007) *Empathy in Patient Care: Antecents, Development, Measurement, and Outcomes*, Springer Science + Business Media, LLC, New York.

Holman, H. and Lorig, K. (2000a) Advances in managing chronic disease, *British Medical Journal* 320: 525–526.

Holman, H. and Lorig, K. (2000b) Patients as partners in managing chronic disease, *British Medical Journal* 320: 526–527.

Joseph, D.H., Griffin, M., Hall, R.F., and Sullivan, E.D. (2001) Peer coaching: An intervention for individuals struggling with diabetes, *The Diabetes Educator* 27: 703–710.

Joshu, C.E. et al. (2007) Integration of a promotora-led self management program into a system of care, *The Diabetes Educator* 33(6 suppl): 151S0158S.

Linn, L.S., DiMatteo, M.R., Cope, D.W., and Robbins, A. (1987) Measuring physicians' humanistic attitudes, values, and behaviors, *Medical Care* 25: 504–515.

Lorig, K., Sobel, D.S., Stewart, A.L., and Brown, B.W. (1999) Evidence suggesting that a chronic disease self management program can improve health status while reducing hospitalization, *Medical Care* 27: 5–14.

Malchodi, C.S., Oncken, C., Dornelas, E.A., and Carmanica, L. (2003) The effects of peer counseling on smoking cessation and reduction, *Obstetric Gynecology* 101: 504–510.

Mensing, C., Boucher, J., Cypress, M., Weinger, K., Mulcahy, K., Barta, P., Hosey, G., Kopher, W., Lasichak, A., Lamb, B., Mangan, M., Norman, J., Tanja, J., Taulk, L., Wisdom, K., Adams, C. (2006) National standards for diabetes self-management education, *Diabetes Care* 29(supplement 1): 578–585.

Miller, W.R. (2009) Ten things that motivational interviewing is not, *Behavioural and Cognitive Psychotherapy* 37: 129–140.

Morgan, J.D. (2002) *Social Support: A Reflection of Humanity*, Baywood Publishing Company, Amityville, NY.

Nettles, A. and Belton, A. (2010) An overview of training curricula for diabetes peer educators, *Family Practice* 27(Suppl 1): i33–i39.

Norris, S.L., Chodhury, F.M., and Van Le, K. (2006) Effectiveness of community health workers in the care of persons with diabetes, *Diabetic Medicine* 23: 544–556.

Norris, S.L., Lau, J., Smith, S.J., Schmidt, C.H., and Engelgau, M.M. (2002) Self-management education for adults with type 2 diabetes, *Diabetes Care* 25(7): 1159–1171.

Paul, G., Smith, S.M., Whitford, D., O'Kelly, F., and Dowd, T. (2007a) Development of a complex intervention to test the effectiveness of peer support in type 2 diabetes, *BMC Health Services Research* 7: 136.

Paul, G., Smith, S.M., Whitford, D., O'Shea, E., O'Kelly, F., and Dowd, T. (2007b) Peer support in type 2 diabetes: A randomized controlled trial in primary care with parallel economic and qualitative analyses. Pilot study and protocol, *BMC Health Services Research* 8: 45.

Peers for Progress. (2010) *Peer Support in Health and Health Care: A Guide to Program Development and Management*, American Academy of Family Physicians Foundation, Tupelo, MS, Leawood, KS.

Philis-Tsimikas, A., Walker, C., Rivard, L., and Talavera, G. (2004a) Improvement in diabetes care of underinsured patients enrolled in project dulce, *Diabetes Care* 27(1): 110–115.

Philis-Tsimikas, A., Walker, C., Rivard, L., Talavera, G., Reimann, J., Salmon, M., and Araujo, R. (2004b) Improvement in diabetes care of underinsured patientes enrolled in project dulce, *Diabetes Care* 27(1): 3.

Piatt, G., Anderson, R.M., Brooks, M.M., Songer, T., Siminerio, L.M., Korytkowski, M.T., and Zgibor, J.C. (2010) 3-year follow-up of clinical and behavioral improvements following a multifaceted diabetes care intervention, *The Diabetes Educator* 36(2): 301–309.

Piatt, G.A., Zgibor, J.C., and Brooks, M.H. (2006) Translating the chronic care model into the community: Results from a randomized controlled trail of a multifacted diabetes care intervention response to Belalcazar and Swank, *Diabetes Care* 29(12): 2762.

Rodriguez, M.S. and Cohen, S. (1998) *Social Support*. In H.S. Friedman (Ed.), Encyclopedia of Mental Health, New York: Academic Press.

Ruggiero, L., Spirito, A., Bond, A., Coustan, D., and McGarvey, S. (1990) Impact of social support and stress on compliance in women with gestational diabetes, *Diabetes Care* 13: 441–443.

Samuel-Hodge, C.D., Headen, S.W., Skelly, A.H., Ingram, A.F., Keyserling, T.C., Jackson, E.J., Ammerman, A.S., and Elasy, T.A. (2000) Influences on day-to-day self-management of type 2 diabetes among African-American women, *Diabetes Care* 23(7): 928–933.

Siminerio, L., Piatt, G., and Zgibor, J. (2005) Implementing the chronic care model for improvements in diabetes care and education in a rural primary care practice, *The Diabetes Educator* 31(2): 225–234.

Siminerio, L.M., Piatt, G.A., Zgibor, J.C., and Emerson, S. (2006a) Deploying the chronic care model to implement and sustain diabetes self-management training programs, *The Diabetes Educator* 32(2): 253–260.

Siminerio, L.M., Piatt, G.A., Zgibor, J.C., and Emerson, S. (2006b) Diabetes self-management education in primary care, *Annals of Family Medicine* 4: 2–3.

Swider, S.M. (2002) Outcome effectiveness of community health workers: An integrative literature review, *Public Health Nursing* 19: 11–20.

Tang, T.S., Funnell, M.M., Gillard, M.L., Nwanko, R., and Heisler, M. (2011a) The development of a pilot training program for peer leaders in diabetes, *The Diabetes Educator* 37(1): 67–77.

Tang, T.S., Funnell, M.M., Noorulla, S., Oh, M., rand Brown, M.B. (2011b) Sustaining short-term improvement rover the long term: Results from a 2 -year diabetes self management (DSMS) intervention, *Diabetes Research and Clinical Practice*, 2012, 95(1), 85–92.

Tang, T.S., Gillard, M.L., and Funnell, M.M. (2005) Developing a new generation of ongoing diabetes self management support interventions (DSMS): A preliminary report, *The Diabetes Educator* 31: 91–97.

Tillotson, L.M. and Smith, M.S. (1996) Locus of control, social support, and adherence to the diabetes regimen, *The Diabetes Educator* 22: 133–139.

Wagner, E.H. (2000) The role of patient care teams in chronic disease management, *British Medical Journal* 320: 569–572.

Wilson, W., Biglan, A., Glasgow, R.E., Toobert, T.J., and Campbell, D.R. (1986) Phychosocial predictors of self-care behaviors (compliance) and glycemic control on non-insulin-dependent diabetes mellitus, *Diabetes Care* 9(6): 614–622.

World Health Organization. (2007) *Peer Support Programmes in Diabetes*, WHO Press, Ed. World Health Organization, Geneva.

10 Diabetes: A Lifetime of Learning

Michelle Robins

Corio Medical Centre, Corio, Victoria, Australia

We have two ears and one tongue so that we would listen more and talk less.
(Diogenes Circa 230–150 or 140 BC)

Introduction

The person with diabetes who knows the most, lives the longest (Joslin 1921, quoted Levetan, 2001). However, the reality nearly one century later, has altered for diabetes educators and is best summed up by William Arthur Ward, scholar, author, editor, pastor and teacher, who said:

Teaching is more than imparting knowledge; it is inspiring change. … Learning is more than absorbing facts; it is acquiring understanding.

Patient education is the cornerstone of diabetes care and education improves glycaemic control (Ellis et al. 2004). Diabetes self-management education (DSME) is defined as the 'ongoing process of facilitating the knowledge, skill, and ability necessary for diabetes self-care' (Funnell 2007, 2010). DSME incorporates a number of components that include needs, goals and the individual's life experiences, all of which are guided by evidence-based practice. The overall objectives of DSME is not just to provide information, but rather to support informed decision-making, effective self-care behaviours, problem-solving skills and actively and collaboratively work with a healthcare team to improve clinical outcomes, health status and quality of life (Funnell 2010).

In 2008, the American Association of Diabetes Educators (AADE) launched the Diabetes Self-Management Education (DSME) Outcomes Continuum. The DSME framework provided the components to measure,

Diabetes Education: Art, Science and Evidence, First Edition. Edited by Trisha Dunning AM.
© 2013 John Wiley & Sons, Ltd. Published 2013 by John Wiley & Sons, Ltd.

monitor and manage diabetes education and its outcomes, but most importantly it emphasised that DSME does not simply focus on the person with diabetes attaining knowledge and skills because these factors do not necessarily influence clinical improvement. DSME provided the educators with the building blocks to alter behaviour that brings change.

The AADE also developed the Seven Self Care Behaviours (AADE7™, Tomky 2008), which is now used in other countries such as Australia. The seven behaviours are seven key steps (behavioural changes) that can improve health and well-being:

1. Healthy eating
2. Being active
3. Monitoring
4. Taking medication
5. Problem-solving
6. Healthy coping
7. Reducing risks (ADEA 2008).

About 40 years ago, Knowles described the principles of adult learning, which are described in Chapter 3. Diabetes educators need to follow these principles when teaching adults with diabetes. However, diabetes educators are far more than 'teachers'; their role includes coaching, motivating, guiding, facilitating, acting as a consultant, negotiating, marketing and counselling.

The phrase 'patient journey' is used, and often misused, to describe clinical pathways and diabetes service models. I use the term to mean the person's emotional, social and physical state at the time of the consultation. For example, questions to consider when using the Flinders Model (2005) may include:

- Are they in shock or denial following the diagnosis of diabetes or the diagnosis of a complication?
- Do they feel having diabetes is unfair?
- Do they attending the appointment intend to bargain over treatment strategies?
  Are they sad or withdrawn and unable to envision a future with diabetes?
- Are they dwelling on the past without diabetes?
- Have they accepted the diagnosis and moved on?

The clinical experience

Diabetes education concerns explaining to people with diabetes why they need to do certain things, not telling them what to do. Likewise, bombarding the person with a barrage of pathophysiological concepts, brochures and handouts and expecting them to make the recommended changes is rarely successful. Ask yourself:

> *Do I really need to know how my car works—the engine, the electrical system, the carburettor, etc., to understand where the petrol and water goes and that I need to have the car serviced regularly? Is it more important for me to drive my car safely and to recognise when it is not working properly and how to get help?*

People can undertake successful diabetes self-management that achieves positive outcomes with a high degree of mastery without knowing diabetes pathophysiology. The educator demonstrates real knowledge and skills when they transform very complex and complicated diabetes information into simple concepts the individual and their family can understand. The art of diabetes education is being adaptable enough to be able to communicate in different ways and styles to suit the individual's needs.

Most people with diabetes are grateful for any information about diabetes self-management. Yet educators must constantly ask themselves: 'Am I really communicating effectively with this person?' The person might nod or answer 'yes' when you asked 'do you understand what I mean?' to please you or not to appear stupid, but such body language does not necessarily convey understanding. Likewise, when a person says 'no' when you ask 'do you have any more questions', they may not actually mean 'no'. Rephrasing the question using different words might evoke a different response.

Educators have a very small window of opportunity to make a real difference in the lives of people with diabetes. Health professionals (HPs) only spend about 0.02% of the time an individual with diabetes lives with their diabetes. HPs expect the individual to perform the seven self-management behaviours the remaining 99.98% of their lives. Thus, diabetes education needs to be dynamic and focused.

One of the biggest mistakes I made when starting out on my journey as a diabetes educator was trying to 'educate' the 'patient' about all aspects of diabetes in the initial consultation. Educators are often under pressure to provide education within a particular session or timeframe. Some educators respond by 'telling' people 'all they need to know about diabetes' in case there are no other education opportunities. Sometimes service systems and health funds limit the number of diabetes education appointments a person with diabetes is entitled to.

Many HPs, including diabetes educators, use 'tick box' assessment tools, which were originally developed to ensure key issues are not overlooked. Although tick boxes elicit information, and fulfil quality management requirements, they largely restrict people to 'yes/no' responses, thus patients and their carers may not be able to share important information that could influence their care plan.

Education 'tick lists' can help newly qualified educators focus the consultation and build their self-confidence until they find their own education style. Tick boxes are not laws written on tablets of stone; they are merely one tool to help educators elicit information. Following them slavishly can result in 'factory line diabetes education' and inhibit the educator's personal and professional growth and development. Adopting a 'one size fits all' approach is one of the greatest mistakes an educator can make.

Many years ago when I was undertaking diabetes educator training, I observed the staff of a highly regarded diabetes education centre that conducted a 6 week individual education programme for people with T2DM. I can still hear a man ask about erectile dysfunction in week 3. He was told that erectile dysfunction would be addressed in week 6, not today. I will never forget the devastated look on the man's face. I could not understand why his question was not answered when it was clearly important to him and he felt comfortable enough to discuss such a sensitive topic with two female HPs. I suspect his question was not addressed at all by week 6. I vowed that, if I were ever lucky enough to work as a diabetes educator, I would never ignore an individual's question. To do so might miss the 'teachable' moment.

Educators teaching Indigenous people develop considerable skills in teaching at teachable moments and eliciting people's stories. One of the first 'rules' educators learn when they engage with Indigenous people is to 'find the story'. In other words, find out what makes the individual tick, how they were diagnosed and the circumstances around the diagnosis, and their life circumstances. Such information is essential, regardless of the individual's diabetes type, age, gender and culture. Individual's social history, home and work situations, and relationships have a direct impact on diabetes self-management, see Chapter 2.

The first question I ask any individual with diabetes, no matter the duration of their diabetes, is: 'did it surprise you when your doctor said you have diabetes?' I do not believe many educators ask the question, yet it yields a great deal of information about the person's beliefs, feelings and often issues that need to be addressed during the appointment. It is quite common for people to state being diagnosed with diabetes came as a surprise and that they were shocked by the diagnosis.

The feeling of disbelief can be so great that the person may not believe they have diabetes, especially if there are no obvious signs or symptoms. It also puts other life events that were occurring at the time of diagnosis, that years later could still be impacting on self-management, into context. Other patients, however, indicate they thought 'something was not quite right' with their health when diagnosed. Sometimes people are 'relieved' to know they have diabetes because they feared they might have 'something worse like cancer'.

Such information can help identify the issues behind denial and questions about whether they really have diabetes. The diabetes educator can explain what the pathology tests mean for the individual and help them identify their diabetes risk factors and how they think they could manage them, or identify whether the diagnosis of diabetes was a catalyst for other life-changing events.

Some older people recently diagnosed with T2DM diabetes, who live a very healthy, active life, maintain a healthy weight and have few other health condition problems, feel particularly upset about being diagnosed with diabetes. Many people believe T2DM is caused by living an unhealthy lifestyle, eating junk food and inactivity. There is a very real stigma associated with T2DM; people in the community and many HPs make value judgments about people with T2DM diabetes. In addition, people with T1DM want clear messages to be promulgated to the community that T1DM is not solely a 'lifestyle disease'.

In Australia one in four people over age 75 has diabetes, often because of increasing age (AusDiab, 2000). It can be useful to focus on the main diabetes risk factor for these people—their age. For example: *'Remember years ago when people got diabetes because of old age, that maybe the pancreas just isn't meant to live to be 100, and maybe it's all due to a bit of wear and tear'.*

An 80-year-old newly diagnosed person with T2DM may not need to make any great changes to their diet, in fact, they have probably followed a 'diabetes diet' for most of their life, thus developed diabetes at 80 instead of age 40. Spending time at the start of a consultation to identify the individual's immediate concerns helps the educator focus the teaching.

Some people regard being diagnosed with diabetes as the end of their world, for example, if they watched someone close to them die from diabetes complications or they remember a family member or friend sharpening needles before they injected their insulin. It is important for the diabetes educator to know such experiences so they do not unknowingly make comments such as: *'well if you don't take diabetes seriously you too could lose a leg and go blind like your mother did'.*

The educator should explain that everyone's diabetes is different and what happens to one individual does not necessarily happen to others. In addition, it is an opportunity to explain and demonstrate modern medications and monitoring equipment and that having T2DM can actually be an opportunity for positive change. For example, *'having type 2 diabetes can actually make you a lot healthier if you're prepared to take on some diabetes self-management'.* People often comment several months, sometimes years later, that being diagnosed with T2DM was the impetus they needed to make the changes in their life and have a healthier and longer life.

However, as mentioned previously, other people are relieved to have diabetes and 'not something worse'. One 60-year-old lady with Latent Autoimmune Diabetes in Adults (LADA) whom I educated was so relieved to learn her weight loss and feeling unwell were due to T1DM and not cancer, particularly bowel cancer, from which her husband died the previous year. She found managing her diabetes, including basal bolus insulin a 'breeze' compared to the chemotherapy her husband had endured.

Some diabetes educators ask people with diabetes whether they have a family history of diabetes. This question will only elicit limited information. Rephrasing the question to ask about the individual and/or *family's* experience of diabetes is more useful. The responses to the two questions are usually very different because the focus is different and the second question is less judgmental. Some people have a family member or a close friend who manages the day-to-day challenges of diabetes and remains well, enjoying the things they like to do, which can be a positive role model. For example:

> *When mum got diabetes, she changed the way she was eating, bought herself a little dog to walk each day, lost weight and really became a much more positive person.*

Other people recall negative experiences, one man said:

> *My dad had type 1 diabetes and it was though the whole family had to have it too, we all had to eat at a certain time and certain foods because of dad's diabetes and we couldn't do the things that other kids did like camping holidays because of dad's diabetes.*

It is important to know the family experience when a person is referred to you to start insulin after 'failing on oral medications'. They might be frightened about injecting insulin because of their family experience. Interestingly, people do not seem to have the same fear about injecting GLP-1 mimetic agents, even though they are afraid of insulin. This anecdotal observation suggests fear is related to insulin rather than needles or having to self-inject. Careful questioning will help distinguish the source of the fear so appropriate education and/or counselling can be provided.

I remember a person with T2DM I taught before insulin pens were available, so he needed to learn how to use a syringe. He had needle phobia. For nearly an hour we discussed his fear of using a syringe and his story changed my approach to insulin-related fear forever. The man's father had T1DM, and when he and his siblings misbehaved, the father chased them around the house brandishing his glass syringe with the needle stabbing at the children as a form of punishment.

Learning styles

Learning theories are outlined in Chapter 3 but a brief outline of teaching and learning styles is presented here. Lifelong learning involves all five senses, sight, speech, hearing, touch and smell, whether the teaching style is active or passive. According to Dunning (2009), learning styles refer to the way an individual acquires, processes, recalls and uses information. Kolb (1984) identified several different learning styles that encompass different learning processes and teaching strategies and noted that a combination of teaching styles are usually needed, especially in group education to cater for a variety of learning styles, see Table 10.1.

Education involves explaining *why* something may or may not work, rather than telling people *what* to do. If you tell a person what to do, they may follow your advice but not understand why or what the benefits are. This means they often stop following your advice because they cannot see the value of continuing. Telling a person why daily activity is important, why insulin is needed, why they need to see a particular specialist makes a difference to their understanding and willingness to continue the behaviour(s). Explanations need to contain a number of elements including the following:

- Being honest and open in your approach.
- Being consistent in the message you convey and use correct terminology and appropriate language (see Chapter 6).
- Simplifying very complex concepts into easier to understand language.
- Determining and building on the individual's existing knowledge base and experience.
- Using catchy phrases, if appropriate and culturally relevant. Rhymes are a good strategy, especially with children.
- Using visual aids.
- Asking the 'right' questions.
- Linking treatment strategies to basic pathophysiology and symptoms.
- Explaining the gaps in our knowledge, research and technology in an understandable way.

Lien at al. (2010) outlined six key points educators need to consider before they begin to teach:

1. Human beings change one behaviour at a time.
2. The key to effective professional/individual interaction is asking good questions and listening to the answers.
3. People respond far more to complements on what aspects of self-management they are achieving or at least attempting, rather than blanket criticism and lecturing.
4. 'Covering the material' and teaching according to rules because 'rules are rules' will not improve clinical outcomes or quality of life.
5. Do not judge people, create a sense of guilt, or threaten patients with potential consequences.
6. A useful first question to ask people is 'what have you heard about taking care of diabetes?'

Table 10.1 Learning styles and some teaching strategies that can be used to facilitate learning.

Learning style	Learning process	Teaching strategy
Active	Retain information by doing something active Like learning in groups Retain information better if they understand it	Teach in group settings Incorporate activities such as demonstrations and return demonstrations Use problem-based learning
Reflective	Prefer to think about things before they act Prefer working alone	Incorporate time for review and reflection Provide short summaries of important information Invite feedback
Sensing	Like learning facts and solving problems using established methods Like details and are good at memorising facts but may do this and not understand the information Like hands on activities Dislike complications and surprises Do not like being asked about information that was not covered in education programmes Practical and careful and like information to be connected to 'the real world'	Show how the information relates to their personal situation and the 'real world' in general Use specific examples
Intuitive	Like to discover possibilities and relationships Like innovation Are bored with repetition Are good at understanding new concepts Usually comfortable with abstract images and statistical information Are innovative and work quickly but may miss important details and make careless mistakes	Link theories to facts
Visual	Remember best when they see pictures, diagrams, flow charts, films and demonstrations	Use visual and verbal information Incorporate concept and mid-maps in the teaching Colour code information, for example 'orange insulin' or 'green insulin' to refer to the package colour
Verbal	Learnt best by listening to words	Use verbal teaching, tapes to take home Group work
Sequential	Learn best if a logical stepwise or staged approach is used May not fully understand the material unless they use it May know a lot about specific topics but have trouble relating them to other aspects of the same subject or to different subjects	Provide logical material where each piece of information follows the preceding information Do not move randomly from topic to topic Give them 'homework' so they can use the information and develop their global learning skills Explain how the information relates to other information

Table 10.1   (*continued*)

Learning style	Learning process	Teaching strategy
Global	Learn large amounts of information without seeing connections and suddenly make the connection May solve complex problems quickly or find innovative ways of doing things once they understand the information May have problems explaining how they did it	Paint the big picture first Explain how topics relate to other topics and to information the person already knows

Be honest

Do not suggest a strategy or course of action you think is inappropriate. You might think a strategy the person wants to try will be ineffective, but give them relevant balanced information, allow them to make the choice and take the responsibility for their decision. It can be helpful to set a time to determine the effects of the individual's choice. For example you could say:

> *Ok let's see what happens when you change your breakfast cereal and type of bread and make a time in four weeks to look at your blood glucose levels again. If your levels are still high we will need to review your diabetes medicines.*

Provide easy to understand explanations about why you believe some strategies will have minimal or a detrimental effect. Using evidence-based information is useful.

Another aspect of honesty is reflection on your own life and more importantly your lifestyle. How healthy is your lifestyle and if it is unhealthy, how much credibility do you have as a diabetes educator? If the person smells cigarette smoke on you and you are suggesting they need to give up smoking, how effective do you think your message will be? Do you eat a healthy diet and do you exercise on a daily basis? If you don't, how convincing will you be when you explain the benefits of these behaviours to people with diabetes? Being a skilled and compassionate educator means 'talking the talk *and* walking the talk'.

Consistent and correct terminology

The words or phrases diabetes educators use can influence self-management (Diabetes Australia 2011). A common inaccurate term is 'blood sugar': there is no such thing as 'blood sugar'. The correct term is 'blood glucose'. You might ask '*Does it matter? It is only semantics after all.*' Yet when a person has hypoglycaemia, the quickest way to increase the blood glucose level is to ingest glucose. Treating hypoglycaemia with sugar takes longer to raise the blood glucose because sucrose and fructose need to be converted to glucose before they can be absorbed into the blood system. Using the phrase 'blood glucose' might help the person with diabetes understand glucose metabolism, the recommended dietary guidelines and glycaemic index.

Likewise, the word 'glucometer' is often used to refer to a blood glucose meter. Glucometer production ceased many years ago, thus most younger people, including community pharmacy staff who sell blood glucose meters, are unfamiliar with such equipment.

Using positive terminology is more than trying to turn a half empty glass into a half full glass. Terms such as 'diet' and 'exercise' have negative connotations for many people regardless of whether they have diabetes or not. Phrases such as 'healthy eating' or 'daily activity' are more positive. Some countries use the word 'shots' to describe insulin injections, but the word has negative connotations in other countries associated with illegal drugs and stigma. 'Injections' or 'doses' might be more appropriate (see Chapters 2 and 6).

Simplifying complex concepts into easier to understand concepts

Diabetes is a very complex range of disorders and we still have a lot to learn about diabetes. T1DM is very different from T2DM. In the latter, a number of key metabolic functions are ineffective. Using familiar metaphors for complex pathophysiology and pathology is useful.

When I discuss changes that could help improve diabetes control, I often mention small changes that people might think are too small to have an impact. These could include the milk used in two cups of tea each day, placing the cooked steak on paper towel to drain more fat from it before eating it, walking a couple laps of the shopping centre before going into the supermarket. I reinforce that these small changes have a cumulative beneficial effect if they are done regularly.

Advanced glycated end products are a very complex clinical phenomenon. However, it can be simplified by describing how hyperglycaemia irritates the lining of large and small blood vessels causing damage that allows circulating fats in the blood to stick onto the lining like *fluff onto Velcro*. It also helps explain why lipid targets are so low for people with diabetes and why most people require statin therapy to reach lipid targets.

Using a car analogy to explain blood glucose is sometimes helpful. For example, glucose is the 'petrol' the body needs, the cells are like a car engine and insulin is like a 'petrol pump'. TIDM has no 'petrol pumps', T2DM does, but they do not work very efficiently. Regular complications screening can also be described as regular 'car servicing' to explain the need for routine complication screening to detect problems early so that they can be treated before they cause too much damage.

I often described nephropathy as being like 'straining spaghetti'. Just like a colander, little holes in the kidneys can widen when blood glucose, blood pressure and lipids are too high, which allows protein from the blood to escape into the urine.

Using the individual's knowledge and experience

As previously mentioned, finding out what makes the individual 'tick' is very important. Information such as their understanding of diabetes, how diabetes fits into their lives and their previous experience of diabetes through family and friends helps the educator plan education and support. It is very helpful to know whether the individual has participated in other health programmes so that you can build on that information. Cardiac rehabilitation group education following surgery represents an opportunity to explain that *'the diabetes diet is very much like the heart diet with less refined sugar in it'*. Being aware of the person's life experiences is a key principle of adult learning.

The reverse is also true; particularly for women with a history of gestational diabetes (GDM) who develop T2DM. These women need to know that the intensity of GDM treatment is different from T2DM management. For example, blood glucose testing will be less frequent, a variety of glucose lowering medicines can be used when a woman is not pregnant and glycaemic targets are less stringent. Many people find the dietary guidelines and recommendations confusing, particularly if they have been given conflicting information by different HPs.

I often ask older people with T2DM what they used to eat when they were 8 years old. If they are unsure how to respond, I describe what I ate when I was 8. We ate a healthy diet with very few 'take away foods' or sweets because of financial constraints, yet it was a balanced diet that met current healthy eating recommendations. I discuss the concept of everyday versus someday foods where soft drink, chips, sweets and chocolate biscuits are the 'someday' foods or irregular treats. Such imagery can help reinforce information they actually know and help them retrieve it from long-term memory stores. Sometimes it comforts older people to know some old ways are better than some new ways.

'Catchy' phrases

Using catchy phrases, often derived from television advertising or slang, can help the educator describe some complex diabetes concepts to people with diabetes and other HPs, provided the target audience understands the slang and the language is culturally relevant and not obscure (see Chapter 6). For example, when informing the individual it might take days or weeks to see a change in blood glucose after starting some medicines, I say *'it's a bit like that shampoo ad, it won't happen overnight but it will happen'*. Many people, especially older men, know the television advertisement and the super model who starred in it! Another example is: *'Hyperglycaemia feels like you are only running on one or two cylinders'*.

When people are in denial, diabetes and its effects, particularly the thought of insulin, can be frightening. Sometimes, people refuse to consider starting insulin despite marked hyperglycaemia and the known health benefits say: *'well you've got to die of something'*. My response is *'well diabetes won't kill you, but the disability from the complications might make you wish you were dead. Think about what it would be like if you have a stroke and you need care in a nursing home to eat your food and use the toilet.'* Some readers will consider this to be a harsh response but reality is also harsh.

When starting a person with T2DM on insulin, I try to 'sell' the idea that it is a fresh start. *'It's not you and what you are eating or doing, but your tablets that are letting the side down, that care coming up short and no longer keeping up their end of the bargain.'* I explain that insulin is has fewer side effects than GLMs and explain that anyone with diabetes, no matter their age, even if they are pregnant, can use insulin safely, that in many ways it is quite a *'natural medication'* helping to boost their own insulin production. The trouble is, injecting is very 'unnatural' for most people.

Sometimes I describe glargine insulin as 'mild' insulin that acts a bit like a 'thermostat' because it does not have a peak action like other insulins. Some people who are extremely fearful of hypoglycaemia find this explanation reassuring. In addition, I focus on the positive changes people make, including having regular pathology investigations, which is an 'insurance policy' for better health. Once I heard low glycaemic index (GI) foods described as low 'human interference' foods, which I found very helpful when discussing breakfast cereals with the people I teach.

Visual aids

A lot of the learning is visual; thus visual images can be very powerful teaching tools. Dietitians have used a variety of visual aids such as food models to illustrate fat on meat, serving sizes, the types of foods recommended, for many years. They use food packages to teach label reading, including teaching during 'supermarket education tours', which makes the learning experience more real than in an office or a health centre.

I have a number of posters in my teaching room that show the different amounts of fat and sugar in certain foods. Most of the people I teach comment on the amount of sugar in orange juice and cola, which is almost identical. I also have an empty 600 mL cola bottle filled with white sugar equal to the amount actually in a 600 mL bottle of coke. Flip charts, diagrams, white boards, dolls, blood vessel models clogged with fat are also useful teaching tools. A combination of written information and pictures is usually more readable than a lot of text, especially if the person has literacy deficits.

When discussing recommended footwear, I ask the individual to take their shoes off and trace their foot on a piece of paper, then place their shoe over their foot trace and describe where the shape of their foot does not fit within the confines of their shoe. This activity is very helpful, particularly for women who persist in wearing shoes that, although stylish, restrict their feet and are potentially harmful.

Asking the right questions

Knowledge is powerful. Knowledge about diabetes and its management is powerful, for the person with diabetes/carers and the educator. Yet, the most knowledgeable diabetes educator may not elicit the relevant or even correct information from a person with diabetes because they do not ask relevant questions, or do not ask them in a way the individual can or will answer.

Asking closed-ended questions elicits limited information and sounds like an interrogation process to the person with diabetes. Asking open questions that require a more detailed response helps the educator acquire the information they need to build a picture of the reality and challenges the individual's life and gives the person a sense of mastery over the education session. The way questions are worded and the association with poor medicine compliance is discussed in Chapter 11. Open-ended questions produce a more honest response than closed questions. Examples of open-ended versus closed-ended questions are shown in Table 10.2.

Many health professionals including diabetes educators use 'tick box' assessment forms. Tick boxes are a good example of closed questions and may not elicit the sort of information that is really useful to understanding an individual's diabetes and their self-management strategies. The ADEA (2010) produced self-management information for people with T2DM that includes a number of questions people should ask HPs about their medicines, including:

- Why am I taking this?
- What effect does it have?
- How does it work?
- When should I take it and how long should I take it for?
- Are there side effects?
- What do I do if I miss a dose?
- What did I do when I'm sick?

Table 10.2   **Example of some alternative ways to ask key questions.**

Instead of asking ...	Try asking ...
What are your results?	What sort of blood glucose levels do you get when you test yourself at home? What do you mean by good? What do you mean by bad?
How often to you test?	When do you test? How long after meals are you testing?
Do you write your results in your diary?	Are there times in your busy day that you miss writing your results in your record book?
Do you wash your hands before testing?	Are you always able to wash your hands before testing? Do you feel comfortable taking your meter with you outside home to use it?
Do you use a new lancet each time?	How many times do you use your lancet before it really starts to hurt? Where on your finger tips are you placing the lancet device?
Have you had your eyes tested in the past 12 months?	When was the last time you had your eyes tested?
Do you have hypos?	How low do your blood glucose levels go?
Do you get symptoms?	How low do your blood glucose levels go before you know it? What sort of symptoms do you have?
How much Novorapid do you take? Do you vary the doses?	In terms of your Novorapid, what sort of doses do you generally take?
Do you miss doses?	What criteria do you use to vary doses, for example, is the dose dependent on your blood glucose level, how much carbohydrate you're about to eat, what sort of activity you intend to do after a meal? Under what circumstances would you not take your Novorapid?

Detailed information about engaging with people with diabetes about their medicines can be found in Chapter 11.

Health literacy

Health literacy is defined as:

> *The degree to which individuals have the capacity to obtain process and understand basic health information and services needed to make appropriate health decisions.*

> US Department of Health and Human Services (2010)

The American Medical Association stated:

> *Poor healthy literacy is a stronger predictor of a person's health than age, income, employment status, education and race.*

Research indicates that inadequate health literacy is independently associated with worse glycaemic control and higher rates of retinopathy in people with T2DM (Schillinger 2002). People with low literacy levels are more likely to

- Be hospitalised
- Stay in hospital longer
- Be unable to comply with recommended treatment
- Make an error with their medications
- Be sicker when they do seek medical attention.

A large Australian adult literacy survey was conducted 2006 that measured the following domains: prose literacy, document literacy, numeracy and problem-solving. Five levels of proficiency were determined, level 1 indicated the lowest level and level 5 the highest literacy level. Level 3 was regarded as the minimum level needed to navigate the demands of everyday life and work.

Forty-eight per cent of women and forty-three per cent of men aged 15–44 years, representing Generations X and Y, who are known for their technical skills and knowledge had a literacy level 3 or above. Literacy level declined markedly with increasing age; only 17% of people aged 65–74 years met the required literacy level. People with sufficient health literacy had more years of formal education, were employed as a professional, earned more than AUS$60 000 per year and were either born in Australia or were English speaking (Australian Bureau of Statistics (ABS) 2006).

More recently, a literacy survey in Adelaide involving 3000 people aged over 15 years found people with inadequate health literacy were more likely to have diabetes, cardiac disease or stroke and were less likely to have recently attended a doctor (Adams et al. 2009). The consequences of inadequate health literacy and the impact on diabetes education are as follows:

1. Health protection; such people are unlikely to be able to:
   a. Read articles in newspapers and magazines
   b. Read health and safety warnings
   c. Know which products to use or avoid
   d. Read information and brochures obtained from HPs and hospital waiting rooms.
2. Disease prevention; such people are unlikely to be able to:
   a. Read alerts on television, radio and newspapers
   b. Read postings about vaccination and screening programmes
   c. Read letters related to test results
   d. Understand graphs and charts
   e. Determine their level of risk and whether to engage in screening, diagnostic tests and follow-up.

3. Systems navigation; such people are unlikely to be able to:
    a. Find out where services are located and what services are available
    b. Understand maps
    c. Fill in application forms
    d. Understand statements of rights and responsibilities
    e. Give informed consent
    f. Understand health benefit packages
    g. Locate relevant facilities.
4. Healthcare maintenance; such people are unlikely to be able to:
    a. Complete health history forms
    b. Read appointment slips
    c. Read medicine labels
    d. Read and follow discharge instructions
    e. Read education booklets and brochures
    f. Find relevant health information on the Internet
    g. Describe symptoms, follow directions on medicine labels, calculate time for medication and collect information about the benefits of different treatments to discuss with HPs.

Thus inadequate health literacy and numeracy directly impacts on diabetes self-management behaviours such as recording self-monitoring blood glucose results, dialling up the correct amount of insulin and understanding the correct number of tablets to take. There is a range of tools HPs can use to measure diabetes-related literacy and numeracy, including the Diabetes Numeracy Test (DNT-15 in both English and Spanish) and the Diabetes Literacy and Numeracy Education Toolkit (DLNET) (White et al. 2010). A systematic review of low literacy and numeracy found that combining individualised teaching and long-term support can help people overcome some of the barriers of low health literacy (Van Scoyoc and De Walt 2010).

Group education

With the increasing number of people developing diabetes, particularly T2DM, diabetes educators are conducting more group education programmes. Group education has several benefits, including developing comradeship, reducing feelings of being 'alone' with diabetes and reassuring people that other people are also trying to make sense of a range of confusing information. Participants ask questions that cover a wide range of issues including questions others had not thought of. People are often able to support each other and share suggestions they find helpful.

Educators can streamline services by creating a pathway whereby several people can receive detailed information from the diabetes team at the same time and reduce waiting lists for individual diabetes educations. However, the facilitator must be expert at facilitating groups, managing group interactions, processes and dynamics (Lowenstein et al. 2009). Lowenstein et al. (2009) identified several requirements of effective groups:

- Fix start and end times.
- Turn mobile phones off.
- State a time limit each person is permitted to speak to enable all group members to participate.
- Establish 'group rules', speaking, for example, raising one's hand before speaking.
- How to refer to each other, i.e. use name and name tags.
- Indicate when breaks will occur and how long they will be.
- Discuss learning contracts such as 'homework'.
- Discuss confidentiality issues.

Structured group programmes improve metabolic control for people with diabetes (Davies et al. 2008; Scain et al. 2009). Traditionally group education was didactic in nature, where the educator delivered information, often using a PowerPoint presentation, which is largely a passive education method. Time was allocated for questions, usually at the end of the session when there was not enough time to adequately answer all questions, the participants had forgotten their question or they wanted to get home.

Sometimes a group is too large to enable effective participant interaction. Some educators discourage questions to ensure they 'keep to the script' and do not run out of time. Often the content focuses on what HPs believe people with diabetes should know, rather than what patients wish to know about self-management and is less likely to result in behaviour change or individual goal setting.

Occasionally people are asked to undertake tasks before the next week's session, which is more likely to identify behaviour that could be modified and the strategies required to do so. For example, they might be asked to set a small goal and when they achieve it, they have the achievement acknowledged by the facilitator and the group.

The DESMOND programme (Diabetes Education and Self-Management for Ongoing and Newly Diagnosed) is delivered in a 6 hour group programme delivered by a multidisciplinary team in either a single day format, two ½ days or three 2 hour sessions. The main of model and learning theories used are the Common Sense Model and Social Learning Theory (Skinner 2006), which showed improved increased understanding of diabetes, the seriousness of diabetes and people's personal responsibility for the 'course'

Table 10.3 **Issues to consider when developing a group education programme.**

Group dynamics	• Group size
	• Type of diabetes, gender, age group, cultural background
	• Access for support person(s) to attend
Group programme	• Topics to be covered and input participates have into information covered
	• Methods of teaching and learning
	• Clinical team members involved with group presentation
	• Handouts provided, level of literacy
	• Time allocated for questions
Specific operational issues	• Day, time, location, does it clash with other activities, for example, shopping on pension day, parking and public transport facilities
	• Costs for clients
	• Do you require formal medical clearance for any exercise component?
	• Promotion of the group via referral pathway, advertising, posted invitations
	• Can people with disabilities or limited English participate?
	• Equipment required
Quality improvement	• How will the group be evaluated?
	• How are participating HPs evaluated?
	• Will people be followed up? If so, how?
	• How will you deal with 'drop-outs'?

of having diabetes. There are many functional and operational issues for the diabetes educator to consider when developing a group education programme (see Table 10.3).

When educating people remember they recall:

- 10% of what they read
- 20% of what they hear
- 30% of what they see
- 50% of what they see and hear
- 70% of what they say
- 90% of what they say and do.

Conversation Maps™ (Healthy Interactions 2009), a series of maps launched throughout the world, address many key factors about T2DM self-management and more recently issues for children with T1DM. The person with diabetes/family members sits around the map on a table. The educator sits on the opposite side of the table looking at the map upside down. Discussion cards and pictures on the maps generate discussion. The facilitator does very little and rarely answers questions. Participants use discussion and problem-solving strategies and most often find the answers themselves.

Sharing personal experiences and changes people made act as a powerful incentive to others. For example, one person complained about the taste of low fat milk. When a dietitian recommends one or two brands that have a similar taste to full fat milk, the individual can be sceptical; however, when another person with diabetes makes that same suggestion, it is a far more powerful message because it came from a person living with diabetes who understands the challenges involved.

The group dictates the direction of each session with minimal direction from the facilitator. Experienced facilitators indicate that the same information is covered in all groups, but the journey varies among groups. This type of programme offers truly person-focused education. Many diabetes educators also use the maps to teach undergraduate nurses, medical and allied health students.

Group education can also be very specific to very specific groups of clients. For example, young adults with T2DM may wish to discuss a range of different issues from older people with T2DM. Targeting specific groups provides an opportunity for people excluded from mainstream group education to participate, for example, people with severe mental illness. Targeting groups with specific needs could assist group dynamics. Age range, socio-economic status and level of education, occupation, life experiences, co-morbidities and geographical location can be so varied in people with diabetes that conducting a 'T2DM' group maybe too 'generic' to enable participants to feel that they have any shared experiences other than diabetes.

Educating people with disabilities

A significant number of people with diabetes have a disability. In 2003, 56% of people with diabetes reported having a disability and one quarter reported that diabetes was the chief cause of their disability occurring (Australian Institute of Health and Welfare 2008). Bainbridge et al. (2008) reported that hearing loss was twice as common in people aged 20–69 years in people with both T1DM and T2DM and that the prevalence of low or mid-frequency hearing impairment was four times high in people aged 20–49 years of age.

Hearing loss appears to be associated with microvascular damage and nerve disease induced by hyperglycaemia in the cochlea. Hearing loss can affect the education. For example, poor hearing may exclude people from participating in group education programmes unless audio education tools or an Auslan translator are available. If they do attend, they usually miss a significant amount of the verbal information provided.

Visual impairment affects all aspects of an individual's self-management, e.g. shopping and cooking, attending appointments, foot hygiene, exercise, medication management and self-monitoring blood glucose. Attending to 'small' details can make a big difference, for example, the colour and font size for PowerPoint presentations and written information, using magnifying sheets when reading labels and magnified fluorescent lamps when performing blood glucose testing. Audio recorded information can be useful (Williams 2009).

Being flexible about where diabetes education is delivered

There is no one best location to provide diabetes education. Education can occur at anytime and anywhere. One of the most challenging locations to provide education is in the hospital when the person is confined to a bed or chair. Wards often offer little privacy, can be loud and noisy and education is interrupted by other staff or visitors. In addition, the individual is often unwell and stressed, all of which can reduce the effectiveness of education provided.

Some educators are located in very convenient addresses such as in or close to a large shopping centre with ample parking and reasonable public transport. Others are located within the GP practice, which may or may not be convenient. Others are employed by large tertiary hospitals with almost no parking or very expensive parking and often long distances for people to walk to the 'diabetes centre' once they find a car park and enter the hospital.

Providing education in a patient's home, especially if they have a disability can relieve the burden and stress generated by attending a clinic. Other people feel they cannot leave their home for education if they are caring for a spouse, for example, with dementia. People prescribed diuretic medication often appreciate afternoon appointments so they can take their medication in the morning and attend an appointment in the afternoon without the stress of looking for a toilet. Dietitians increasingly provide education in supermarkets. Supermarket tours were discussed earlier in the chapter.

Playing DVDs in waiting rooms can help reinforce lifestyle messages and self-management strategies. Electronic education formats are increasingly available and are discussed in Chapter 12. A variety of mobile phone apps are available to assist people count carbohydrates and adjust insulin doses. The 'virtual' diabetes educator is emerging.

Cultural sensitivity and diabetes education

Increasing cultural diversity represents new challenges for diabetes educators (Jack 2007). Health beliefs differ considerably among different cultures and impacts on health behaviours and self-care. Organisations and diabetes educators need to be culturally sensitive and increase their knowledge and understanding of how diabetes is perceived and treated in different cultures how to sensitively deliver education.

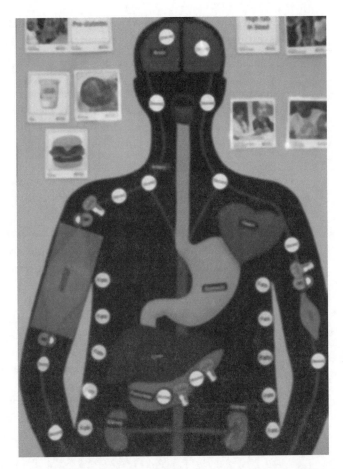

Figure 10.1 "The Feltman" teaching tool for indigenous clients. Feltman is a resource developed by Diabetes Australia-Victoria and the Victorian Aboriginal Community Controlled Health Organisation (VACCHO) and produced with funding from the National Diabetes Services Scheme. The National Diabetes Services Scheme is an initiative of the Australian Government administered by Diabetes Australia. (Reproduced with permission from Diabetes Australia.)

Simply translating Anglo-Saxon dietary advice into another language does not take account of different foods and cooking methods. For example, translating breakfast cereal from English into Vietnamese is inappropriate, because many Vietnamese people living in Australia do not eat cereal for breakfast. Some women from Muslim backgrounds consider exercise unfeminine and unacceptable. Other cultures use herbal or Chinese medicines and regard using them as very positive and proactive approach to diabetes self-management (see Chapter 11). The 'Feltman' (see Figure 10.1) is a teaching tool widely used during education with Indigenous people, it is culturally sensitive and meaningful for participants.

Cultures that regularly fast also require additional support to minimise risks during fasting times, e.g. Ramadan. The AADE (2007) defined cultural sensitivity as:

The extent to which ethnic/cultural characteristics, experiences norms, values, behavioural patterns, and beliefs of a target population's relevant historical, environmental, and social forces are incorporated in the design, delivery, and evaluation of targets health promotion materials and program.

The AADE listed a number of strategies to consider when providing diabetes education to a people from different cultural backgrounds:

- Become familiar with cultural variations in families, health beliefs, patterns of community practice, for example how different religious periods can affect an individual's decision to access a health service or undertake pathology testing.
- Respect different cultural health beliefs.
- Engage and collaborate with different cultural groups and promote the use or development of health workers from specific groups.
- Review and research the different relationships between culture, health and diabetes in order to develop new or revised therapeutic approaches to improving diabetes care.
- Develop learning materials in partnership with specific cultural groups.
- Be aware of certain behaviours exhibited by the diabetes educator that may be viewed as inappropriate or disrespectful to some patients, for example touching and eye contact.

Be aware of language

Language is a powerful tool; in fact Rudyard Kipling said *'words are, of course, the most powerful drug used by mankind'*. In 2011 Diabetes Australia released a Position Statement acknowledging the importance of language that highlighted the impact of inappropriate language (Diabetes Australia 2011). Language is explored in detail in Chapter 6.

Where to start

With so many different learning theories, approaches and strategies, it is difficult to determine which approach will be the most effective for each individual. Dunning (2009) developed a simple tool that could help identify people's dominant learning style. The tool can easily be incorporated into routine education and care (see Table 10.4).

Table 10.4   **Dunning (2009) brief tool to assess learning style.**

Please put a number in the line in the order that best describes how you learn new important information.
Number 1 is the way you learn best and 10 the way you learn least effectively
If you choose the 'other' option please briefly describe what you do to learn new information

1. Read printed information such as books and pamphlets with a lot of words
2. Read printed information with lots of pictures and diagrams or see models of things
3. Watch videos/DVDs, television, YouTube clips
4. Listen to an audiotape, radio talkback, podcast or a lecture
5. Have someone show you how to do a task such as blood glucose testing
6. Talk with other people who have similar problems:
   a. In a group
   b. In an Internet chat room
   c. Individual information discussion
7. Practise using equipment such as injecting insulin or cooking food
8. Other, please specify

The tool has not been validated and people with vision and literacy deficits may need assistance to complete the tool.

Chapter summary and key points

What and the way diabetes educators teach should be constantly refined. Diabetes educators need to reflect on how they teach and the outcomes of their interactions with patients and their families. Educators need to be open to new ideas and actively seek feedback from peers and people with diabetes. Finding time to observe colleagues is an important part of this process. Sharing strategies and ideas is vital.

Key points:

- Education is life long for people with diabetes, their family or significant others and HPs.
- Education should be tailored to the individual needs including their learning styles, health literacy level, health beliefs and experiences, cultural background, presence of disability and goals for self-management.
- Attaining knowledge in itself is not the main focus or outcome of health education. The aim is to help the individual change or develop health behaviours beneficial for diabetes self-management and contribute to improved health outcomes.
- Communication is the key to providing quality education.
- Education is provided in 'chunks' rather than trying to cram every aspect of self-management into a session.
- Quality education is about identifying what the person wants to know rather than purely the agenda of the diabetes educator.
- Sometimes concepts need to be 'unlearnt' first before new learning can occur.
- Myths, misinformation and outdated concepts are derived from the Internet and well-meaning friends/family members and need to be addressed.

- Education can be conducted in a variety of ways and in combination ranging from individual appointments to group education in a variety of locations.
- Changing a health behaviour is often not related to health itself, but assisting in a different goal identified by the person with diabetes.
- The ultimate goal is that life should get in the way of diabetes, rather than diabetes get in the way of life.
- Brochures do not replace diabetes education.

Reflective questions

Reflection is a key part of the person with diabetes' journey: it is equally important for HPs to reflect on their journey as an HP and educator. The following are some questions you might like to reflect on. It sometimes helps if you think about a person with diabetes you educated recently and felt you did not do the job as well as you would like to.

- How much listening do you do when educating people and their families with diabetes?
- Do you practise active listening?
- Have you asked a colleague to observe and critique your interactions with people with diabetes?
- Do you observe how peers conduct education sessions with people with diabetes as a learning opportunity?
- Do you readily seek feedback from the team about how you could implement other therapeutic approaches with people who exhibit challenging behaviour?

References

American Association of Diabetes Educators AADE7™. (2007) Self-care behaviors. http://www.diabeteseducator.org/ProfessionalResources/AADE7/

AusDiab Report Diabesity and Associated Disorders in Australia.(2000) The Accelerating Epidemic. The Australian Diabetes, Obesity and Lifestyle Study http://www.bakeridi.edu.au/Assets/Files/AusDiab_Report_2000.pdf (accessed September 2011)

Australian Bureau of Statistics Adult Literacy and Life Skill Survey. (2006) http://www.ausstats.abs.gov.au/ausstats/subscriber.nsf/LookupAttach/410 2.0Publication30.06.093/$File/41020_Healthliteracy.pdf (accessed August 2011)

Australian Diabetes Educators Association (ADEA). (2008) Diabetes self care: The 7 steps to success. Canberra, ADEA.

Australian Diabetes Educators Association (ADEA). (2010) Looking after your type 2 diabetes: Smart steps. Canberra, ADEA.

Australian Institute of Health and Welfare. (2008) Diabetes Australian Facts 2008.

Bainbridge, K., Hoffman, H., Cowie, C. (2008) Diabetes and hearing impairment in the United States: Audiometric evidence from the National Health and Nutrition Examination Survey 1999–2004. *Annals of Internal Medicine* 149(1):1–10.

Davies, M., Heller, S., Skinner, R. et al. (2008) Effectiveness of the diabetes education and self management for ongoing and newly diagnosed (DESMOND) program for people with newly diagnosed type 2 diabetes: Cluster randomized controlled trial. *British Medial Journal* 336(7642):491–495.

Diabetes Australia. (2011) Position Statement: A new language for diabetes, improving communications with and about people with diabetes http:// www.diabetesaustralia.com.au/PageFiles/18417/11.09.20%20DA%20 position%20statement.pdf

Dunning, T. (2009) *Care of People with Diabetes: A Manual of Nursing Practice* (3rd edn.). Chichester, Wiley-Blackwell.

Ellis, S., Speroff, T., Dittus, R., Brown, A., Pichert, J., Elasy, T. (2004) Diabetes patient education: A meta-analysis and meta-regression. *Patient Education and Counseling* 52:97–105.

Flinders Human Behaviour and Health Research Unit, *Chronic Condition Self-Management Education and Training Manual*. Flinders University, January 2005.

Funnell, M. (2010) National standards for diabetes self-management education. *Diabetes Care* 33(suppl 1):s89–s96.

Funnell, M., Anderson, R., Austin, A., Gillespie, S. (2007) AADE position statement individualization of diabetes self-management education. *Diabetes Educator* 33(1):45–49.

Healthy Interactions. (2009) The US Diabetes Conversation Map® Program http:// www.healthyinteractions.com/conversation-map-programs/ conversation-map-experience/current-programs/usdiabetes

Jack, L. (2007) AADE position statement cultural sensitivity and diabetes education: Recommendations for diabetes educators. *Diabetes Educator* 33(1):41–44.

Kolb, D. (1984) Cited in Arndt, M. and Underwood, R. (1990) Learning style theory and patient education. *Journal of Continuing Education in Nursing* 21(1):28–31.

Levetan C. (2001) Adding a daily dosage of diabetes wisdom to your prescription. *Diabetes Spectrum* 14(3): 163–167.

Lien, L., Cox, M., Fenglos, M., Corsino, L. (Eds.) (2010) *Glycemic Control in the Hospitalized Patient*. New York, Springer.

Lowenstein, A., Foord-May, L., Romano, J. (2009) *Teaching Strategies for Health Education and Health Promotion: Working with Patients, Families and Communities*. Sudbury, MA, Jones and Bartlett Publishers.

Scain, S., Friedman, R., Gross, J. (2009) A structured education programs improves metabolic control in patients with type 2 diabetes: A randomized controlled trial. *Diabetes Educator* 35(4):603–611.

Skinner, T. (2006) Diabetes education and self-management for ongoing and newly diagnosed (DESMOND): Process modeling of pilot study. *Patient Education and Counseling* 64:369–377.

Tomky, D. (2008) AADE position statement AADE7™ self-care behaviours. *Diabetes Educator* 34(3):445–449.

Van Scoyoc, R., De Walt, D. (2010) Interventions to improve diabetes outcomes for people with low literacy and numeracy: A systematic literature review. *Diabetes Spectrum* 23(4):228–237.

White, R., Wolff, K., Cavanaugh, K., Rothman, R. (2010) Addressing health literacy and numeracy to improve diabetes education and care. *Diabetes Spectrum* 23(4):238–243.

Williams, D. (2009) Making diabetes education accessible for people with visual impairment. *Diabetes Educator* 35(4):612–621.

11 Medicine Self-Management: More than Just Taking Pills

Trisha Dunning AM

Deakin University and Barwon Health, Geelong, Victoria, Australia

> *We chat together, sire; he gives me prescriptions;*
> *I never follow them, so I get well.*
>
> Molière quoted in Taschereau (1822)

Introduction

Medicines are central to most people with diabetes' care plan. The purpose of this chapter is to explore people with diabetes' medicine-related beliefs and behaviours, not to discuss the pharmacodynamics and pharmacokinetics of medicines or how to choose a medicine regimen. Such information can be found in most medicine formularies and diabetes textbooks. Health professionals (HPs) can have a significant effect on people's medicine self-management practices, which can be positive and affirming or negative and disempowering. The latter is more likely to lead to medicine non-compliance and less than optimal outcomes. HPs also have their own medicine-related beliefs and behaviours, which are shaped by their experiences just as people with diabetes' experiences shape their beliefs and behaviours.

Although a healthy diet and regular activity are essential, most people with diabetes need medicines to manage or prevent hyperglycaemia, hypertension and lipid abnormalities as well as to treat other concomitant conditions. The cost of uncontrolled diabetes is high for both the individual and society, thus metabolic targets have become more stringent since the release of the findings of the Diabetes Control and Complications Trial (DCCT) (1993) and the United Kingdom Prospective Study (UKPDS) (1998). It is now common for people with T2DM to take three to four antihypertensive agents, oral glucose lowering medicines (GLM) and/or

Diabetes Education: Art, Science and Evidence, First Edition. Edited by Trisha Dunning AM.
© 2013 John Wiley & Sons, Ltd. Published 2013 by John Wiley & Sons, Ltd.

insulin: usually more than one GLM and more than one insulin type, lipid-lowering agents as well as other medicines.

Dunning and Manias (2005) found people with diabetes took an average of 7.4 medicines per day, range from 1 to 12 in multiple doses at various times during the day, which is polypharmacy. There are several definitions of polypharmacy, and the term may have different meanings and be understood differently in different populations. For the purpose of this book polypharmacy was defined as:

> *The use of a number of different drugs* [medicines] *possibly prescribed by different doctors and often filled in different pharmacies, by a patient who may have one or several health problems.*
>
> Mosby's Medical Dictionary (2009)

Some researchers refer to 'thoughtful' and 'unthoughtful' polypharmacy to distinguish between careful considered medicine combinations and an *ad hoc* process of adding medicines to the existing medicine regimen, which often occurs when multiple prescribers are involved. Polypharmacy in diabetes could be thoughtful polypharmacy to comply with recommendations in medicine titration algorithms and guidelines because it addresses the multifactorial metabolic and other abnormalities associated with diabetes. However, to be truly thoughtful, the effects on the individual, including the 'pill burden', must be part of the decision-making framework. In addition, polypharmacy can only be truly thoughtful if the person with diabetes is actively involved in medicine-management decisions.

Medicines are associated with a high rate of errors, adverse events (AEs) and hospital admissions (Green et al. 2007; Jenkins and Vaida 2007). Medicine errors and AEs also occur *in* hospitals and aged-care facilities and result inconsiderable morbidity and mortality (Roughead and Lexchin 2006). Importantly, many errors and AEs are avoidable (Jenkins and Vaida 2007). Box 11.1 outlines some of the factors associated with medicine-related errors and AEs.

Significantly, some medicines commonly used to manage diabetes, such as insulin, are regarded as high-risk medicines (HRM) because they have a high risk of causing harm, even when they are used as prescribed (Institute of Safe Medicine Practice 2008). Children, pregnant women and older people are particularly vulnerable groups and are at greater risk of AEs. A number of strategies have been implemented to reduce medicine-related errors and AEs (see Box 11.2).

Medicine self-management

Inappropriate medicine use affects health outcomes such as blood glucose, lipids and blood pressure. Medicine self-management is complex and

Box 11.1   Overview of some of the factors associated with medicine-related errors and adverse events

- Older people; for example, 30% of unplanned hospital admissions of older people are associated with medicine errors or AEs. A number of factors are involved: changed medicine pharmacokinetics and pharmacodynamics due to the ageing process and renal and liver disease, which can alter medicine metabolism and excretion and can lead to accumulated doses. In addition, medicine self-management can be compromised by mental, visual, fine motor skills and problem-solving deficits. This means older people are at risk of Type A AEs, which are largely predictable, thus, many could be prevented. Some older people rely on family and other carers to help them manage their medicines, which adds another layer of complexity to the medicine error potential
- People with serious health conditions who use multiple medicines, for example using 5 or more regular per day and more than 12 doses per day
- People using medicines with a narrow therapeutic index, which are usually high-risk medicines (HRMs) such as insulin, heparin, cancer medicines and opioids
- Recent transitions between care facilities, for example between hospital, rehabilitation or age care facilities and home
- Discharge from hospital within the preceding 4 weeks
- When changes to the medication regimen are not recorded on discharge summaries or communicated among relevant healthcare providers
- When people consult a number of HPs, some of whom might be CAM practitioners
- Changes in the treatment regimen within the preceding 3 months
- People using complementary medicines (CAM) and other CAM therapies, especially if they do not disclose their use and when CAM use is not documented
- People with literacy and numeracy deficits
- Administering medicines via the wrong route
- When HPs transcribe medicine prescriptions, e.g. telephone medicine orders
- Distractions during medicine administration rounds

(Newman 2010), The Australian Institute of Health and Welfare (AIHW) (2009); Stowasser et al. (2004); The Australian Commission on Safety and Quality in Healthcare (2010). The last three are health professional-related.

Box 11.2   Evidence-based strategies and processes used to reduce medicine-related errors

- Proactively identifying people at risk of non-compliance and being aware of the factors associated with non-compliance
- Using quality use of medicines, which encompasses using non-medicine options where possible and stopping unnecessary medicines, i.e. reducing polypharmacy
- A range of medicine safety standards and guidelines, e.g. Australian National Commission on Safety and Quality in Health Care, UK Department of Health and the US Institute of Safe Medicine Practice standards
- Computerised Physician Order Entry programme
- A range of clinical decision support tools
- Automated alert systems that alert HPs to the need to ask the individual about medicine allergies. Another form of alerts, HRM medicine alerts, alert HPs to the problems associate with HRM and suggest strategies for reducing the risk. The latter may not reach all key stakeholders
- Educating HPs and people with diabetes and carers about medicine-related errors and how to reduce them. Medicine alerts can trigger education for HPs but were not designed for the public. However, education needs to be interactive, use a range of strategies and link the information to relevant local and individual issues
- Ward-based pharmacists and other strategies where pharmacists, doctors and nurses work closely together, e.g. on medication safety committees and medicine review programmes
- Regular comprehensive medicine reviews and medicine reconciliation programmes for people most at risk, e.g. those described in Box 11.3. Six monthly medicine reviews might be indicated for older people prescribed more than four medicines
- Using a structured validation processes in hospitals and aged-care homes when prescribing and administering high doses of insulin, e.g. > 50 units of intermediating acting and mixed insulin and > 25 units of short or rapid acting insulin. Only having 50 unit syringes available for general use on the wards also reduces high dose insulin errors
- Improving communication among HPs and with people with diabetes and carers, and discharge planning

Rommers et al. (2007); Wolfstadt et al. (2008); Dooley et al. (2011); Fowler and Rayman (2010); National Heart Foundation of Australia (2011).

requires the individual to master complex medicine-specific self-care behaviours. Medicine self-management is far more complex than 'taking the medicine as directed', yet people are often labelled non-compliant if they do not follow HP advice.

> *I got a new medicine script from my doctor three months ago but I don't know what to do with it. He told me to take it three times a day but by the time I got to the chemist I forgot what he said and I could not understand the chemist lady because she had an accent—Chinese, I think. Anyway I didn't want to stay there asking questions because she started talking louder when I asked her about taking it [medicine] so I left. I'm not deaf, you know. Then I tried to read the label on the box but the print is so small and it just said take one tablet three times a day as directed, but I do not know what that means so I decided not to take them, anyway they are pretty big and look hard to swallow. It's all too much bother so I don't take it.*

This lady's decision could be construed as non-compliance—but is it? Was it common sense? Perhaps her non-compliance actually prevented a medicine-related error, AE or admission to hospital. It is impossible to tell without understanding her general, cultural, health and medicine-related beliefs. Certainly it appears she did not have the information she needed to make an informed decision about her new medicine. Her story also shows some of the people involved in the 'medication pathway' who need to give clear, specific, consistent information, clearly did not—so who was non-compliant within their respective roles? What role did the doctor and the pharmacist play in the lady's decision to not take the medicine?

Many people do not understand directions such as 'take one tablet three times a day' for various reasons, including inadequate literacy and numeracy skills and the fact that such information is ambivalent and unclear (Davis et al. 2009). People need clear, explicit directions about how to manage their medicines. The lady's experience highlights the fact that people do not receive the medicine information they need to manage medicines safely, even when HPs explain medicines to them (Dunning and Manias 2005).

Complementary and alternative medicines and therapies

Complementary and alternative medicines and therapies (CAM) use is very common: more than 50% of the population in most countries use CAM. Many people with diabetes use CAM medicines and other CAM (Egede et al. 2002; Dunning 2003; Manya et al. 2012). People, especially older people, also use over-the-counter medicines such as analgesics (Roumie and Griffin 2004). CAM use can be self-initiated or an HP might refer the individual to a CAM practitioner. People with diabetes use CAM for a number of reasons including to improve well-being and quality of life, manage pain, stress and intercurrent illness such as colds and 'flu', to treat unpleasant symptoms including medicine side effects, and because they encompass spirituality 'they treat the whole person'.

Purposeful (thoughtful) CAM use, whether CAM is used alone or in combination with other medicines and treatments, has risks and benefits. At the very least, HPs must ask about CAM use in a non-judgemental way and document it. In addition, people need education about safe CAM use, just as they need information about other medicines. A knowledgeable HP must supply CAM information, and this might not be a conventional HP. In addition, conventional practitioners need to rethink the contention that CAM GLM 'do not work'. Some do, as the following story shows.

A 26-year-old Chinese lady who recently returned from visiting her mother in China was being investigated for an insulinoma because she was having frequent episodes of profound hypoglycaemia. Her mother had T2DM and had just been diagnosed with cancer. Tests demonstrated very high plasma insulin levels that correlated with very low plasma glucose and hypoglycaemia symptoms but radiological investigation did not identify the site of the insulinoma. The lady was scheduled for exploratory surgery to locate the insulinoma.

I asked the doctors

have you asked Miss XX whether she has been using any CAM medicines.
Yes—she said no.
What words did you use when you discussed it with her?
I asked if she was using any unproven or alternative treatments.
Do you mind if I talk with her about CAM and her visit to her mother in China?
Go ahead.

There were three important clues that Miss XX's hypoglycaemia could be due to herbal GLM: being Chinese, her recent visit to China and her mother's T2DM. When I asked her about her visit to China and how her mother was getting on she said:

> Mum was more worried about me making the long trip home when my work is so busy. She thought I looked tired and had no energy so she gave me some of her diabetes medicines to increase my energy levels. That's when I started having these turns, but I kept taking the medicine to increase my yang. She got them from the Chinese medicine doctor.

The story shows the importance of using appropriate language when asking questions, being non-judgemental, considering cultural issues and having an open mind.

'Compliance': to use or not to use, that is the question

Although I rarely, if ever, ask people with diabetes about 'compliance', I choose to use 'compliance' rather than adherence or concordance or other euphemisms in this chapter, even though the recently released Language Position Statement (Diabetes Australia 2011) stated compliance can have negative connotations for people with diabetes. One reason I choose to use compliance is that it is difficult to find one agreed definition of compliance and the word is used interchangeably with other words such as adherence and concordance. The three words, compliance, adherence and concordance, do not actually mean the same thing and all three have both positive and negative connotations. Some authors use compliance to refer to shared decisions between the individual and the HP prescriber: a positive connotation (Segal 2007; Bissonnette 2008).

The main reason I choose compliance is that it is actually a composite term that includes three interrelated concepts:

1. Acceptance, which refers to the individual's informed choice to use medicines to improve or maintain their health (World Health Organisation (WHO) 2003).
2. Adherence, which encompasses the degree to which the individual follows agreed medicine regimens (Cramer et al. 2007), that is, adopts appropriate medicine self-management.
3. Persistence, which refers to the duration of using the medicine from the time it is commenced to the time it is discontinued (Cramer et al. 2007). Some medicines such as insulin in T1DM are required for life; thus, we do not expect the person with T1DM to stop taking insulin, even temporarily. In fact many non-diabetes HPs need to be reminded that insulin should not be stopped in T1DM even for short periods of time because it increases the risk of ketoacidosis. Short courses may be required for self-limiting illness, for example, antibiotics. People prescribed antibiotics are often told they 'must complete the full course', yet most people stop the antibiotics when they feel better. Some infectious diseases specialists now believe it is not necessary to complete the full antibiotic course. Thus, stopping antibiotics before completing the prescribed course may not be non-compliance and could reduce medicine costs and the impact of antibiotic overuse on resistant organisms. The same might apply to other medicines prescribed for a specific time course.

In order to reach an agreement, or make a shared decision, both parties need access to and be able to understand relevant information about the various management options. The HP needs to understand the individual's medicine beliefs and attitudes and behaviours. If such an agreement cannot be reached, and maintained, the desired outcome is unlikely to be achieved (Cramer et al. 2007). Often the HP's perspectives and those of the person with diabetes are different, and they have different ways of determining benefit and risk (see Chapters 3 and 4) (Britten 2003). Another consideration is whether 100% compliance (optimal compliance) is required or whether an individually determined 'appropriate' compliance rate is acceptable. The latter often happens, for example stopping antibiotics when feeling better.

However, optimal compliance is important with some medicines such as those with a narrow therapeutic index such as digoxin, warfarin and insulin in T1DM to main therapeutic blood levels. Thus, desired outcomes and compliance must be examined from at least two perspectives: the person with diabetes and the HP, and sometimes other people involved in medicine management such as family caring for children and older people. In some cases, dispensers (pharmacist) and funder perspectives might need to be considered.

People with diabetes' perspective

Understanding the person with diabetes' perspective is essential to enable the HP help them decide on a medicine self-care regimen that suits their lifestyle and achieves the desired mental and physical outcomes. People with diabetes consider several factors when deciding to take/not take a medicine and considering the benefits and risks of medicines. Some factors include the following:

- Cost: some people reduce doses or change dose intervals to reduce costs even though many medicines are subsidised in Australia, e.g. *'We're good mates. We've all got the diabetes and we do lots of things together and we all pretty much take the same medicines. So we decided to pool our medicines when we get 'em from the chemist and share 'em out. Sometimes we run out before we can get more, but we do pretty well'* (Dunning and Manias 2005). Underuse of medicines because of cost is a problem in many countries (Kemp et al. 2011).

- Likelihood and type of side effects: e.g. *'I will not take any more of those satin medicines* [statins] *they make me ache. The doctor said I was imaging things, but it is me that's aching and I know when I'm aching and I don't want to ache.'* Likewise, some people with diabetes reduce insulin doses to avoid hypoglycaemia, a common and significant side effect of insulin and sulphonylureas. HPs do not always recognise or understand the effects of hypoglycaemia on well-being, the fear it engenders and the associated sense of loss of control and sense of vulnerability. (Tay et al. 2001).

- Remembering to take the medicines in their usual daily routines. People with diabetes in the Dunning and Manias (2005) study gave a range of reasons for forgetting to take their medicines for a range of reasons. Most did not worry about the missed doses and took the next due dose; others took all or part of the dose when they remembered. For example:

- *'I'm getting old and my memory—well she ain't what she used to be you know.'*
- *'I always forget my insulin at work because I get busy and distracted. I'm just too busy sometimes, well often actually.'* This man's story illustrates competing priorities the individual needs to accommodate.
- *'I never forget my metformin but I often forget my insulin.'*
- *'I am not sure I really forget to take them—I just take a rest from them when I am on holidays and when I eat out. That's not the problem for me; I have trouble remembering to take them when the holiday is over.'*
- Perception that taking medicines means 'you are sick'. *'I won't take insulin it means you have come to the end of the road—it is the last resort and I have no options left. No I won't take it'* (Dunning 1998).
- Stigma associated with injecting insulin in public because *'they might think I am a drug addict'*.
- Whether they can *'stop the medicine for a while sometimes, you know have a little holiday from medicines'*.
- Medicine burden (polypharmacy) *'I am on so many medicines and each time I see another specialist for all my problems they give me another one. It is hard to remember to take this one before meals and this one after meals and the little green one, I call it rat sack, must be swallowed whole. But I have a system now for taking it in turns to stop some of them for a while. I don't feel any different when I do so I think it is a good system.'*
- Cultural customs and beliefs: for example, Chinese people avoid situations and times likely to bring bad luck and often avoid visiting a doctor or going to hospital on certain days, especially Chinese New Year, and many do not take medicines at this time (Yen Yang et al. 2011). Interestingly, Yen Yang is a Taiwan national interviewing Chinese people with diabetes who immigrated to Australia about their diabetes self-care practices; she did not find this practice unusual because it is *'just part of my culture'*. However, it was important interesting information for Rasmussen and I (co-researchers) because we are from a different culture.

Strictly speaking, many of these quotes illustrate non-compliance: they also provide a great deal of insight into how and why people make decisions about using/not using medicines. In addition, considering the positive aspects, they also reflect proactive decision-making, albeit the decisions may not be ideal from an HP's perspective. They make a great deal of sense if we consider the individual experiences embodied in the quotes and reflect on how common they are—if HPs only ask!

It is also important to point out that the individuals disclosed the information during routine diabetes outpatient clinic consultations and interviews conducted as part of medicine-related research. In both settings, non-judgemental questions, active listening and acceptance were employed to establish a trusting relationship with the individual. These techniques helped the individuals feel safe to disclose information about their behaviours most knew HPs usually regard as non-compliance.

The accuracy of self-reported behaviour is problematic. However, research suggests people who say they do not follow treatments usually report accurately, but those who report they follow treatment recommendations usually report inaccurately (Spector 1986).

HPs, especially prescribers and educators perspectives

HPs generally base their decision to recommend a medicine and decide doses and the dose regimens on the following:

- An assessment that encompasses physical, and hopefully, emotional aspects but does not always include exploring the individual's medicine perspectives or capability in any detail, often because of time constraints.
- Prescriber's previous experience managing diabetes and its treatment. For example, registrars often adopt similar practices to the consultants with whom they trained. However, there is evidence that physician compliance with care standards decrease as physicians become more experienced and that older physicians are less likely to adopt newly 'proven' therapies (Choudhry and Fletcher 2005). It is not clear whether the same is true for other HPs groups. Likewise, a number of reasons could account for the finding.
- Decision-making aides such as online medicine handbooks and diabetes guidelines. These guidelines include the recommendation to achieve normoglycaemia and control lipids and hypertension to prevent diabetes complications.
- Information gained from pharmaceutical representatives, continuing medical education programmes and conferences.
- Their understanding of the individual's beliefs and ability to afford medicines.
- Concerns about multiple prescribers being involved and the risks associated with inadequate communication among prescribers and dispensers.

Carers, particularly family members

Carers often assume a care role when the individual is too young, has mental and/or physical disabilities or is no longer able to self-care because of age-related disabilities. Parents usually receive information, but it is not always the case with older people. For example, we found that husbands and wives caring for their relatives with diabetes receiving palliative care were very distressed and unsure about their knowledge and ability to help their relative with diabetes perform self-care activities such as injecting insulin and blood glucose monitoring (Dunning et al. 2012).

Developing a trusting partnership with carers is essential and might include providing accurate, timely and easy to understand medicine education. In fact, Carer's Australia would like general practitioners to include a 'carer identification field' on their professional electronic software packages such as prescribing and e-Health programmes (Hughes 2010).

HPs need to appreciate that carers provide support and care for older relatives with complex needs. The carers are often also old and have health problems and may require medicines themselves. The stress of caring for an older relative may mean they neglect their own health and may not 'take their medicines as directed'. Thus, carers might need education about their relative's medicines as well as their own medicine regimen and advice about how to accommodate medicines management into their other personal and care-giving responsibilities.

Carers are also an important source of information and can provide valuable information about their relative's medicine history, beliefs and behaviours that might not otherwise be available.

Extent of non-compliance

Many researchers have explored medicine compliance, but although they often use different definitions of compliance, there is clear evidence that non-compliance is common. People are reluctant to take medicines, even modern medicines with fewer side effects, and try to reduce the number of medicines they take (Pound et al. 2005). Common ways of measuring compliance include:

- Pill counts.
- Frequency of completing the full course of a medicine.
- Prescription refill rates.
- MEMs containers, which have a microprocessor in the lid that records the data and time the container is opened. MEMs do not measure actual use. They are expensive, even for research purposes. The theory is that if a person opens the medicine container, they are likely to take the medicine.
- Self-reported medicine behaviours using self-completed questionnaires, interviews or informal discussing during clinical consultations (Matsuyama et al. 1993; Kriev et al. 1999; Dunning and Manias 2005; Cramer et al. 2007).

These studies indicate dose omissions, stopping medications without consulting an HP and inappropriately changing medicine doses are common.

Haynes et al. (1996) found half the medicines prescribed for chronic diseases are not taken. Other research suggests one fifth of people do not begin to take prescribed medicines (e.g. the lady on page 181), a further fifth stop taking medicines before they complete the full course and a further 40% do not take their medicines 'as directed'. Many of these examples of 'non-compliance' are evident in the quotes on page 185.

Adjusting medicine doses is interesting. HPs expect insulin-treated people with diabetes to eventually learn how to and to adjust their insulin doses according to their blood glucose patterns, activity, diet and illness. Thus, an individual who practises insulin dose adjustment is actually undertaking appropriate medicine self-management and most likely preventing AEs. Not adjusting insulin doses could be non-compliance in some circumstances such as during illness because it can result in ketoacidosis, a serious life-threatening condition.

Is there a relationship between medicine compliance and optimal health outcomes?

If people do not take their medicines, they will not 'work'. However, there is a complex relationship between people's compliance rates (optimal, appropriate or not appropriate) and the effects on health outcomes, but understanding about the relationship is limited. One reason for lack of information is the different ways outcomes are measured and the fact that most measurement tools are subjective (individual self-reports such as the quotes in this chapter) or objective, valid scales (Di Matteo et al. 2002). Likewise, many randomised controlled trials that examine medicine efficacy do not consider compliance in the study design.

Despite these limitations, compliance has a positive effect on treatment outcomes (Di Matteo et al. 2002; Simpson et al. 2006). Di Matteo et al. (2002) undertook a meta-analysis of 63 studies and found compliance reduced the risk of no or poor outcomes by 26% compared with non-compliance. The DCCT (1993) and UKPDS (1998) demonstrated improvements in HbA_{1c} and other parameters, which were partly due to medicines although it is possible some of the effects could be attributed to regular monitoring, support and encouragement from the research team.

A number of other factors affect the outcomes. These include the pharmacodynamics of the particular prescribed medicines, which is affected by a number of individual factors such as age, gender and pharmacogenetics. Factors that induce the enzymes involved in medicine metabolism result in shorter duration and intensity of the medicine effect. Factors that inhibit the enzymes have the opposite effect. Enterohepatic circulation, intestinal flora and nutrition status play a role.

Likewise, altering medicine dose forms can affect the duration of action and medicine bioavailability, for example, crushing long-acting dose

Box 11.3   **Risk factors that *could* indicate an individual is at risk of medicine non-compliance and needs to be assessed**

- Outcomes are not as expected, e.g. fall in HbA_{1c}, lipid, blood pressure or the response is not as great as expected
- Prescriptions not filled
- Missing appointments especially after a recent hospital admission
- Appear forgetful, cognitively impaired, distressed or depressed
- Difficult life situation
- Develop a new problem, which could be a medicine side effect, e.g. nausea or bloating with metformin or hypoglycaemia with insulin and sulphonylureas. Alternatively, it could be a complication of diabetes
- Have multiple co-morbidities associated with difficulty performing usual activities of daily living including opening medicine containers, vision or hearing deficits, which can result in social isolation
- When there are few symptoms, e.g. MI, foot ulcers and UTI
- When the person does not accept the diagnosis of diabetes
- Inadequate social support or a carer who also has health and/or mental problems
- Low income
- Inadequate coping, problem-solving, self-esteem and interpersonal skill, which might result in social withdrawal
- Literacy and numeracy deficits
- Do not believe the medicine will be beneficial and the medicines are not aligned with cultural or individual health beliefs
- Dissatisfied with the treatment options
- People who are travelling or working in shifts
- Unable or unwilling to answer questions about their medicines
- People who report they miss doses, inappropriately adjust doses or stop medicines

The more risk factors present, the more likely the individual is to be non-compliant. However, the presence of these risk factors does not mean the individual is not taking their medicines. As indicated, factors other than the person with diabetes' compliance influence medicine-related outcomes.

forms of metformin and inappropriately cutting medicines in half because of cost.

Identifying people at risk of non-compliance can and should par part of the HP's medicine-management role (Australian Council on Quality and Safety in Healthcare 2002, 2010). Yet, doctors did not detect 57.1% of non-compliance in one study (Bieszk et al. 2003). Do nurses and educators do any better? Box 11.3 outlines some of the main risk factors for medicine non-compliance.

Factors that influence medicine compliance

Many factors influence medicine compliance including:

- Whether HPs not proactively monitor and identify people at risk of non-compliance and importantly, medicine errors and AEs.
- Individual characteristics such as age, beliefs, physical and mental capability, social situation, literacy and numeracy levels, problem-solving skills, living alone, support available and medicine knowledge. There is some evidence that women with arthritis may be more compliant than men (Viller et al. 1999), but it is not clear whether this also applies to women with diabetes.
- '*I just forget*'. Remembering or forgetting to take medicines is an individual characteristic. It is normal to forget sometimes and there are many causes including cognitive deficits that could indicate dementia states but this also occurs during hyper- and hypoglycaemia and temporarily affects memory, decision-making and problem-solving capacity, and depression and anxiety states (see Chapter 2).
- Presence of diabetes complications and concomitant conditions. This is also an individual characteristic, which can make medicine-related tasks such as opening medicine containers especially those with child-proof lids, dividing tablets in half (if appropriate) and testing blood glucose difficult. Such conditions include vision impairment, hearing deficits and conditions that affect fine motor skills such as arthritis.
- Medicine regimen such as dose frequency and the number of medicines. Polypharmacy was discussed on page 180.
- Medicine availability and cost where people often stop medicines or find creative ways to accommodate medicine costs such as the medicine 'sharing co-operative' the group mates developed (page 184).
- The HP–individual relationship. People who have a good relationship with their doctors are more likely to comply (Kerse et al. 2004) (see Chapter 3).

How is compliance assessed/measured?

Compliance is difficult to measure because many aspects of compliance are intangible: however, a variety of tools are used, which can make it difficult to compare study outcomes. Some experts recommend measuring continuous rather than dichotomous or ranked variables and suggest several methods should be used, including self-report. It is obvious from the quotes used in this chapter that people's stories yield vital information relevant to the individual that would only be captured using open questions and self-report formats.

The information in people's stories is vitally important to planning care and achieving optimal outcomes for the particular individual, but may be irrelevant to other people. However, such stories occur in all cultures. The inaccuracy of self-reported information, including HPs, is acknowledged. It occurs for various reasons such as forgetfulness, wanting to 'save face' and wanting to please the HP.

There is no 'gold standard' way to measure compliance. The choice of measurement tools will depend on whether data are collected for research, in which case it will depend on the research question, or whether the purpose is to measure individual clinical outcomes. In both cases, a combination of methods is likely to yield the 'best' data. Some commonly used research methods were described on page 187. Research and clinical monitoring also includes:

1. Physiological markers such as HbA_{1c}, blood glucose and lipids, blood pressure and medicines, and blood and/or urine levels. Presence or absence of symptoms, e.g. pain, thirst and polyuria indicating hyperglycaemia and angina.
2. Clinical judgement based on physical assessment, observation.
3. Self-report, e.g. people might volunteer information, keep diaries/record books of their medicines use in their blood glucose record book.
4. Australian Pharmacy Guild Adherence Monitoring System, Medsindex, which compares actual and expected prescription refills according to the dose regimen (Pharmacy Guild of Australia 2010).
5. Scales such as:
    a. Brief Medicines questionnaire (BMQ)
    b. Morisky Scale
    c. Medicines Adherence Report Scale (MARS)
    d. Beliefs about Medicines Questionnaire (BaMQ)

The Morisky scale is widely used despite the fact it has limited validity and uses judgemental language. For example, one question asks: 'Are you careless at times about taking your medicines?'

Strategies that can help people with diabetes use their medicines safely and effectively:

Fewer than 50% of strategies used to improve medicine compliance are effective (World health Organisation (WHO) 2003). As indicated, the HP–individual relationship makes a significant difference to compliance and safe medicine use. Therapeutic relationship is discussed in more detail in Chapter 3. Multiple, individualised strategies that involve actively discussing medicines with the person with diabetes, including the factors that make it difficult/easier to comply, and providing the information the individual needs in a format that suits their learning style are key strategies (Williams et al. 2008).

Note these strategies are HP-related and include:

● Reflecting on their medicine-related beliefs and behaviours and whether they achieve optimal compliance.

- Engaging people with diabetes and carers in conversations about medicines self-management using an open neutral conversation style, choosing words carefully and avoiding ambiguity, for example: *'You are on a lot of medicines, how do you remember to take so many?'* Listening to the words and the way the individual uses words is very helpful to knowing how to phrase information and questions (see Chapter 6).
- Employing quality use of medicines (QUM) to selecting medicine options.
- Maintaining own medicine knowledge and competence.
- Effectively communicating with colleagues and people with diabetes and carers.
- Competently using medicine-related technology.
- Understanding the risk factors for and indicators of non-compliance and proactively assessing people for these factors (see Box 11.4).
- Providing appropriate medicine education. Box 11.4 suggests some key information people with diabetes and carers need to manage their medicine self-management plan. Such information can be conveyed in a number of ways. Consumer Medicines Information (CMI) is used in some countries to facilitate discussion, but the information may be too complex for many people with diabetes, especially those with literacy and numeracy deficits.
- Recommending memory aids such as dose aids/organisers and dose reminders, mobile telephone alarms and other prompts.
- Undertaking comprehensive medicine reviews including in the individual's home. Although pharmacists conduct medicine reviews, other HPs have a responsibility to be involved in the process, at the very least recognise the need for a review. It is important to take a medicine history as well as document the medicine regimen. For example, the following true story illustrates two very different medicine experiences for the same person that affected medicine-related beliefs and behaviours differently.

My first recollection of having medicine was when mum took me for my vaccinations before I started school. She explained that it would be a needle and it would probably hurt but the doctor had lots of practice giving needles. She also told me she would not be upset if I needed to cry. The needle hurt. I did not cry. Mum gave me a big cuddle, told me she knew it hurt and how brave I was, and bought me a new book. This was a very positive, affirming experience.

I was in my 30s when I had my next encounter with a medicine and it was horrific. I was prescribed an antibiotic for a serious infection. I developed excruciating abdominal pain and symptoms suggesting I had a bowel obstruction. I was being prepared for an emergency laparotomy when my GP suggested it could be pseudomembraneous colitis due to the antibiotic. It was. The GP saved me from surgery. But not from vowing I will never take and antibiotic again. I use CAM instead.

Box 11.4   Some information about medicines that can help people with diabetes use their medicines safely and effectively

- The name of the medicine, preferably the name of the active ingredient in the medicine rather than the brand name. People need to realise it is important to know the name of the active ingredient and the difference between the name of the active ingredient and the brand name
- Explain what generic medicines are
- The reason the person needs the medicine (what it is for)
- How the medicine works
- When to take it; for example, when to take insulin and GLMs in relation to food and exercise
- How to take it
- How to store it. Some people may need information about storage and handling during travel
- Side effects and the *individual's* likelihood of experiencing such side effects. How to recognise a side effect and what to do if they experience a side effect
- Special precautions if any apply, for example interactions with foods and other medicines
- How to read the medicine label. There are 22 types of labels and 14 types of additional label instructions in Australia formulated for specific purposes. Labels also contain information about the incipients and fillers in medicines. Some people are allergic to these and some to the colourants in medicines. Labels also should have the expiry date, manufacturing information and batch number
- Tallman lettering can be helpful if medicines have similar names
- Appropriate disposal of unused medicines and related equipment
- Some people might need hints to help them remember to take their medicines and what to do if they miss a dose or doses
- Some medicines will be prescribed for a specific time period. People need to know when and how to stop taking such medicines
- Whom to contact for advice
- How to determine a reliable Internet medicines information site that conforms to the Hon Code (http://www.healthconnect.org/HONcode?conduct.html accessed October 2011)

Written information should use clear, unambiguous language and be specific. Design layout, colour contrast, font size and font type all influence the acceptability and readability of written information.

- Organising peer medicine education programmes. The Council for The Aging collaborates on such programmes in Australia (Hughes 2011). Peer education is discussed in Chapter 9.

Quality use of medicines

QUM emphasises the central role of the consumer in safe medicines use (Figure 11.1). It is a useful framework for thinking about medicines because it encompasses the following:

- Regulatory processes such as approving medicines for use as well as manufacturing, labelling, marketing, and storing and disposing medicines.
- Practitioners using appropriate assessment processes to determine whether medicines are required.
- Recommending non-medicine options where possible and if appropriate.
- Selecting and prescribing appropriate medicines, medicine doses, formulations and duration of treatment if a medicine is indicated and reviewing the patient's response.
- Monitoring and reporting medicine errors and AEs, and applying the learning gained from such events to improve practice.
- Educating medicine users/carers about optimal medicines use, storage and disposal.
- Communicating effectively among HPs and medicine users (Commonwealth Department of Health and Ageing 2002).

QUM, diabetes educators and medicine management

Medicines are used in five main areas of diabetes care and thus the educator's practice:

1. **Primary prevention** where lifestyle factors and prevention programmes avoid/delay the need for medicines. However, medicines often have a preventative role for people with diabetes, for example lipid-lowering and antihypertensive medicines.
2. **Secondary prevention** where medicines are used to prevent or treat diabetes complications and/or other co-morbidities.
3. **Clinical care** to actively treat the metabolic abnormalities associated with diabetes and its complications.
4. **Documenting and communicating** relevant information to other HPs and the individual and their carers. Such information could include management goals, triggers for medication review or cessation, AEs and medication self-management information. Communicating

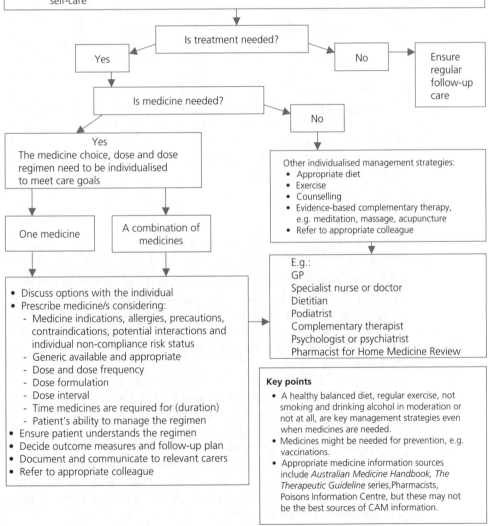

Figure 11.1 **A quality use of medicines (QUM) framework for managing medicines.**

medicine information is particularly important when the individual makes transitions among health providers and services.

5. **Research and clinical trials** where clinical medicine trials are a standard way of investigating medicines. Research is used to develop clinical practice guidelines, position statements and information for HPs and people with diabetes/carers.

Summary

Medicine self-management is complex and challenging. HPs can play a key role helping people with diabetes manage their medicines appropriately by engaging with the individual to determine and understand their beliefs about and experience of medicines, which will help put their medicine-related behaviours into perspective. Compliance and non-compliance are accepted HP terminology. They are descriptors that might mean different things to people with diabetes and their carers. However, the terms should not be used as judgemental labels.

I thought carefully about using the terms 'take', 'use' and 'administer' to refer to the act of 'taking a medicine'. I used 'take' and 'use' interchangeably to be consistent with the literature. To me, take refers to oral routes, use can refer to any route, as can administer, but the latter sounds more like an HP word. One rarely hears a person with diabetes say 'I administered my insulin'.

Reflective questions

Reflection is essential to learning. It is a key part of the person with diabetes' journey and it is equally important for HPs to reflect on their journey as carers and educators. The following statements or questions may help you reflect. It sometimes helps if you think about a recent encounter with a person with diabetes where you felt the encounter did not go as well as you would like.

- Recall a personal medicine experience you had. Was it a positive experience or was it a negative experience?
- How did you feel at the time?
- How did it affect your beliefs about medicines?
- How did it affect your subsequent medicine-related behaviours?
- A particular view about compliance and non-compliance was described in this chapter. How do you feel about the terms compliance and non-compliance?

References

Australian Commission on Safety and Quality in Healthcare (ACSQHC). (2011) *National Safety and Quality Health Service Standards*. ACSQHC, Canberra, pp. 34–39.

Australian Council on Quality and Safety in Healthcare (ACSQHC). (2002) *Second National Report on Patient Safety—Improving Medication Safety*. ACSQHC, Canberra.

Australian Council on Quality and Safety in Healthcare. (2010) http://www.health.gov.au/internet/safety/publishing.nsf/Content/NIMC_005_Medication-Safety-Alerts (accessed May 2010).

Australian Institute of Health and Welfare (AIHW). (2009) *Australian Hospital Statistics 2007–2008*. AIHW, Canberra.

Bieszk N, Patel R, Heaberlin A. (2003) Detection of medication non-adherence through review of pharmacy claims data. *American Journal Health Systems Pharmacy* 15(60):360–366.

Bissonnette J. (2008) Adherence: A concept analysis. *Journal Advanced Nursing* 63(6):634–643.

Britten N. (2003) Commentary: Does a prescribed treatment match a patient's priorities? *British Medical Journal* 327:840.

Choudhry N, Fletcher R. (2005) Systematic review: The relationship between clinical experience and quality of health care. *Annals of Internal Medicine* 144:260–273.

Claydon-Platt K, Manias E, Dunning T. (2011) Development of the diabetes medication risk screening tool to identify people with diabetes at increased risk of medicine-related problems. *British Journal of Clinical Pharmacology* (under review).

Commonwealth Department of Health and Aging. (2002) The quality use of medicines. Commonwealth Department of Health and Aging, Canberra.

Cramer J, Roy A, Burrell A, Fairchild C, Fuldeore M, Ollendorf D, Wong P. (2007) International Society for Pharmacoeconomics for Outcomes Research Working Group. Medication compliance and persistence: Terminology and definitions. *Value in Health* 11(1):4447.

Crystal D. (2006) The fight for English: How language pundits ate, shot and left. *Babel* 44(2): 39.

Davis T, Federman A, Bass P, Jackson R, Middlebrooks M, Parker R. (2009) Improving patient understanding of prescription drug label instructions. *Journal General Internal Medicine* 24:57–62.

Diabetes Australia (DA). (2011) *A New Language for Diabetes: Improving Communication with and About People with Diabetes*. DA, Canberra.

Diabetes Control and Complications Trial Research Group. (1993) The effect of intensive treatment of diabetes on the progression of long term complications of insulin dependent diabetes. *New England Journal of Medicine* 329:977–986.

Di Matteo M, Giordani P, Lepper H, Croghan T. (2002) Patient adherence and medical treatment outcomes: A meta-analysis. *Medical Care* 40(9):794–811.

Dooley M, Wiseman M, McRae A, Murray D, Van De Vreede M, Topliss D, Poole S, Wyatt S, Newnham H. (2011) Reducing potentially fatal errors associated with high doses of insulin: A successful multifaceted multidisciplinary prevention strategy. *British Medical Journal* 20:637–644, doi:10.1136/bmjqs.2010.049668 (accessed December 2011).

Dunning T. (1998) *How Serious is Diabetes: Perceptions of Patients and Health Professionals*. PhD thesis, Deakin University Library, Melbourne.

Dunning T. (2003) Complementary therapies and diabetes. *Complementary Therapies in Nursing and Midwifery* 9:74–80.

Dunning T, Manias E. (2005) Medication knowledge and self-management by people with type 2 diabetes. *Australian Journal of Advanced Nursing* 11:172–181.

Dunning T, Savage S, Duggan N, Martin P. (2012) The experiences and care preferences of people with diabetes at the end of life. *Journal of Hospice and Palliative Care Nursing* 14(4):293–302.

Egede L, Xiaobou Y, Zheng D, Silverstein M. (2002) The prevalence and pattern of complementary and alternative medicine use in individuals with diabetes. *Diabetes Care* 25:324–329.

Fowler D, Rayman G. (2010) Safe and effective use of insulin in hospitalised patients. http://www.diabetes.nhs.uk/document.php?o=1040 (accessed January 2011). National Health Service, London.

Gilbert A, Roughead L, Sanson L. (2002) I've missed a dose: What should I do? *Australian Prescriber* 25(1):16–18.

Green J, Hawley J, Rask K. (2007) Is the number of prescribing physicians an independent risk factor for adverse drug events in an elderly outpatient population? *American Journal of Geriatric Pharmacotherapy* 5(1):31–39.

Haynes R, McKibbon A, Kanani R. (1996) Systematic review of randomised trials of interventions to assist patients to follow prescriptions for medications. *Lancet* 348:383–386.

Hughes J. (2011) Carers' role in the quality use of medicines. Presented at *National Medicine Symposium*, 26–28th May. Melbourne Convention Centre, Melbourne, p. 67.

Institute of Safe Medicine Practice (ISMP). (2008) High risk medicines. www.ismp.org (accessed January 2011).

Jenkins R, Vaida A. (2007) Simple strategies to avoid medication errors. http://www.aafp.org/fpm/2007/0200p41.html (accessed December 2009). AAFP, Leawood, KS.

Kemp A, Roughead E, Preen D, Semmens J. (2011) Determinants of self-reported medicine underuse due to cost in Australia and six other countries. Presented at *National Medicine Symposium*, 26–28th May. Melbourne Convention Centre, Melbourne, p. 82.

Kerse N, Buetow S, Mainous A, Young G, Coster G, Arroll B. (2004) Physician-patient relationship and medication compliance: A primary care investigation. *Annals of Family Medicine* 2(5):455–461.

Krauss R, Fussell SR. (1991) Perspective-taking in communication: Representations of others' knowledge in reference. *Social Cognition* 9: 2–24.

Kriev B, Parker R, Grayson D, Byrd G. (1999) Effect of diabetes education on glucose control. *Journal Louisiana State Medical Society* 151(2): 86–92.

Manya K, Champion B, Dunning T. (2012) The use of complementary and alternative medicine among people living with diabetes in Sydney. *BMC Complementary and Alternative Medicine* 12:2, doi:10.1166/1472-6882-12-2

Matsuyama J, Mason B, Jue S. (1993): Pharmacy interventions using an electronic med-event monitoring device: Adherence data versus pill count. *Annals of Pharmacology* 27(7–8): 851–855.

Mosby. (2009) *Mosby's Medical Dictionary*, 8th edn. Elsevier, Amsterdam.

National Heart Foundation of Australia (NHFA). (2011) *Improving Adherence in Cardiovascular Care*. NHFA, Canberra.

Newman B. (2010) Safety first. *Nursing Review* June 2010: 26.

Pound P, Bitten N, Morgan M, Yardley L, Pope C, Daker-White G, Campbell R. (2005) Resisting medicines: A synthesis of qualitative studies of medicine taking. *Social Science and Medicine* 61: 133–155.

Rommers M, Teepe-Twiss I, Guchelaar H-J. (2007) Preventing adverse drug events in hospital practice: An overview. *Pharmacepidemiology and Drug Safety* 16: 1129–1135.

Roughead E, Lexchin J. (2006) Adverse drug events: Counting s not enough, action is needed. *Medical Journal of Australia* 184(7): 315–316.

Roumie C, Griffin M. (2004) Over-the-counter analgesics in older adults—A call for improved labeling and consumer education. *Drugs and Aging* 21: 485–498.

Segal J. (2007) 'Compliance' to 'Concordance': A critical view. *Journal of Medical Humanities* 28: 81–96.

Simpson S, Eurich d, Radjeedp S, Ross I, Varney J, Johnson J. (2006) A meta-analysis of the association between adherence to drug therapy and mortality. *British Medical Journal* 333: 15–18.

Spector P. (1986) Perceived control by employees: A meta-analysis of studies concerning autonomy and participation at work. *Human Relations* 39: 1005–1016.

Stowasser D, Allison Y, O'Leary K. (2004) Understanding the medicine management pathway. *Journal of Pharmacology Practice Research* 34: 293–296.

Taschereau J. (1822) *Histoire de la vie et des overages de Molière, 1825*. Paris. Translated in: *The North American Review* 27: 60, [New Series 18: 35]. Boston, MA, p. 386.

Tay M, Messersmith R, Large D. (2001) What do people on insulin therapy remember about safety advice? *Journal of Diabetes Nursing* 5(6): 188–191.

The Pharmacy Guild of Australia. (2010) Medindex: A medicine compliance indicator. Http://www.medsindex.com.au (accessed November 2011). The Pharmacy Guild of Australia, Canberra.

United Kingdom Prospective Study (UKPDS 33, 34). (1998) Intensive blood glucose control. *Lancet* 352: 837–853, 854–865.

Viller F, Guillemin F, Briancon S, Moum T, Suurmeijer T, van den Heuvel W. (1999) Compliance to drug treatment of patients with rheumatoid arthritis: A 3 year longitudinal study. *Journal of Rheumatology* (26): 2114–2122.

Williams A, Manias E, Walker R. (2008) Interventions to improve medication adherence in people with multiple chronic conditions: A systematic review. *Journal of Advance Nursing* 63(2): 132–143.

Wolfstadt J, Gurwitz J, Field T, Lee M, Kalkar S, Wu W, Rochon P. (2008) The effect of computerized physician order entry and clinical decision support on the rates of adverse drug events: A systematic review. *Journal of General Internal Medicine* 23(4): 451–458.

World Health Organisation (WHO). (2003) *Adherence to Long-Term Therapies: Evidence for Action*. WHO, Geneva.

Yen Yang, Dunning T, Rasmussen B. (2011) Chinese people's experience of diabetes self-care in Australia. *Diabetes Conquest* Summer: 9–10.

12 The Advance of Health Information Technology: Travelling the Internet Superhighway

Kari Harno

LKT Dosentti FHIMSS, Kerava, Finland

If a group of people don't already share knowledge, don't already have plenty of contact, don't already understand what insight and information will be useful to each other, information technology is not likely to create it.

Introduction

The diabetes nurse educator requires technologies to support day-to-day activities and to successfully reach patient-focused behavioural objectives. Although use of technologies in health is pervasive, it may soon become ubiquitous. This chapter outlines current uses of healthcare information technology (HIT) and technological solutions the diabetes nurse educator will need in the near future for education, management and self-care of their patients.

Internet and networks

Although present day information technology (IT) owes its existence to converged Victorian-era inventions, the telegraph and telephone, weaving the Web into a superhighway arises as a unique feat comparable to Gutenberg's press, Bell's telephone and Marconi's radio. We envision the superhighway as an environment where most citizens walk. At the same time, many people fear that technology is dehumanising us by taking away creative aspects of personality, or compassion and sensitivity towards others, but Michael Dertouzos elegantly phrased that technology

Diabetes Education: Art, Science and Evidence, First Edition. Edited by Trisha Dunning AM.
© 2013 John Wiley & Sons, Ltd. Published 2013 by John Wiley & Sons, Ltd.

is an inseparable child of humanity and for true progress to occur the two must walk hand in hand (Berners-Lee 2000).

The exchange of information in networks before the Web thrived on a decentralised technical, as well as social, architecture. Web 1.0 allows users to retrieve information, but linking all the information stored in computers everywhere will not find the solution to our problems, although the Web is capable of performing the bulk of the legwork required. Tim Berners-Lee, the creator of this Web, pointed out that information retrieval gets things done faster, but exhausts us in the process. Therefore, reaching desired goals will not emerge spontaneously from information abundance, although diabetes educators become more competent and citizens empowered through access to a much wider range of information.

Learning is a remarkably social process and information is only one of the pieces in creating progress. Documents do not merely carry information, but enable virtual communities among those who share information to reach common understanding and new concepts. Since traditional communities have mostly declined, networks may develop a sense of belonging if they can create an image of the group as a single community.

Web 2.0 sites allow users to do more than just retrieve information by providing the user with a platform for community collaboration by blogs and wikis. Facebook aptly describes its social dimension and these forms of cooperation, provided that privacy is protected by encrypted communication and secure identification, may apply for multidisciplinary working groups and interactions with diabetics. Because citizens have changed more than the organisations on which they depend, these new working models could tailor services individually according to personalised need.

What the social media models are enabling is decentralised individual communication (Mezrich 2010). The ability to create and update content leads to the collaborative work of many rather than just a few. This paradigm will allow people to get more of their information through constant updating in this network. Another approach to be provided by the semantic Web (Web 3.0) is driving the evolution of the current Web and allowing users not only to find, share and combine information more easily, but also enable data on the Web to be located and processed automatically on behalf of the user.

As we seem to be naturally built to interact with others, it is necessary to identify that this reciprocity takes various forms. Two types of work-related networks, with the boundaries they inevitably create, are critical for understanding learning, work and the movement of knowledge (Brown and Duguid 2002). First, there are the networks that link people to others whom they may never get to know but who work on similar practices or are amalgamated by shared caring for diabetics. These are the 'networks of practices' and they are notable for their reach, which may be fortified by information technology. Although these networks produce little new explicit knowledge, they are operationally very efficient in supplementing tacit and collective learning to this process. Scaling and outsourcing of services, driven and supported partly by developments in IT, has become established policy in many countries multiplying the complexity of these service networks.

Second, there are the more tight-knit groups formed, again through practice, by people working together on the same or similar tasks. These are what we call 'communities of practice'. Here coordination is tight, and ideas and knowledge are distributed in productive and innovative fashion. While information technology and information sharing is very good in reach, it may suit less well to the dense interaction already in place between practices in the same unit.

Diabetes education

Patient-focused chronic care means that healthcare is organised to maximise the effectiveness of patients to manage their chronic illness themselves. Effective and efficient methods of management, particularly in home care and community-based services, have been devised that enhance the ability of patients with chronic care to participate in their healthcare (Holman and Lorig 2000). Three programmes place patients in a central role in their healthcare—self-management education, group visits and remote medical management.

Educational programmes have become an integral part of diabetes care, but despite the fact that comprehensive implementation of diabetes education remains an outstanding unmet need (Grusser 2011), HIT has not been applied in self-management education to a greater extent as catalyst for successful diabetes therapy. Providing information to patients for dealing with medical management, emotional management and role management is insufficient on its own to improve clinical outcomes (Murray 2008a). Paradoxically at times, the patient may appear 'more informed', especially if their condition is chronic as in diabetes. This may arouse defensible reactions (legitimate and appropriate) from professionals towards the exploitation of HIT.

Besides acquiring knowledge and skills as outcomes of diabetes self-management education, behaviour changes such as developing confidence, motivation and problem-solving skills to perform self-care and overcome barriers have been adopted for effectiveness of diabetes education (Mulcahy et al. 2003). The role of HIT may be partly seen in essence as a support and enabler of lifestyle and behaviour management of the diabetic by the following:

- Health information services that provide general and specific information and guidance (http://www.nhs.uk/Pages/HomePage.aspx, http://ndep.nih.gov/, http://www.ndei.org/)
- Peer communities for interaction among citizens or patients about shared health concerns; a form of social media (http://www.peersforprogress.org/about_us.php)

Several objectives, extending from commercial incentives to academic motivation, exist when diabetes education material is made available on the Web. The problem is no longer finding information but assessing the credibility of the publisher as well as the relevance and accuracy of a document retrieved from the Net. Content has to be appropriate and evaluated to the intended need. A site sponsored or facilitated by a product supplier does not necessarily provide a balanced view. Also the date of last update and the credentials of the authors require judgement prior to use.

The principles documented by the Health on the Net Foundation (HON) state 'that health-related websites must make clear the sources which they have used and ensure that the information presented is appropriate, independent and timely. As some sites may be sponsored by one party and hosted by a different one, these relationships should be clearly disclosed on the site'. The HONcode has been accredited to over 5500 sites and 1, 2 million web pages (http://www.hon.ch/med.html). The web site includes user guidance tools to guide in the review of health web sites.

A chronic disease self-management programme, for example the NHS expert patient programme, is facilitated by a lay leader and aims to enhance the self-efficacy to manage health (http://www.expertpatients. co.uk/course-participants/courses/expert-patients-programme). These, and other similar programmes, have a positive effect on participants' self-efficacy, but disappointingly small effect on health outcomes, quality of life and healthcare use (Eysenbach et al. 2004; Foster et al. 2007). An alternative may be Internet-delivered health interventions. Although more research is needed on how such interventions work, who they work for and for what conditions, preliminary data suggest they can be effective under some conditions (Murray 2008b). Peer education harnesses the power of social norms by enabling people to spread health messages through their social networks (Campbell et al. 2008).

Coaching develops patients' skills in preparing for a consultation, deliberating about options and implementing change (O'Connor et al. 2008). It may be provided face-to-face (FTF), or over the telephone, email or Internet. Health coaches are most commonly found in call centres, which improves access and coverage but usually lacks continuity or linkage with primary care practices. Linkage to care may make it easier to identify and tailor the coaching to the patients' needs. Coaching needs to be tailored to individuals and integrated with existing health systems.

A systematic review assessed the evidence on implementing change. Motivational interviewing draws on people's need for cognitive consistency. The combined effects of 72 trials of motivational interviewing in patients with various diseases showed no effect on glycated haemoglobin values, but significant positive effects were found for body mass index, total blood cholesterol and systolic blood pressure (Rubak et al. 2005). HIT applications for nascent use in motivational interviewing have only recently been initiated.

Provider technology

- *Electronic health record (EHR)*
- *Diabetes registry*
- *Clinical decision support (CDSS)*

Patient technology

- *Personal risk assessment tools*
- *Self-management tools*
- *Remote monitoring*
- *Personal health record (PHR)*
- *Patient decision support (PDSS)*

Figure 12.1 **Overview of current health IT technologies used by healthcare providers or people with diabetes. Provider technologies represent comprehensive care applications in chronic care. Data are captured by professionals and information stored securely within the organisations. Patient applications support self-care management and enable diabetics to capture and review their own data, which may be shared with a third party over the Internet.**

Less patient facing technology is in use today than HIT in healthcare organisations (Figure 12.1), but there appears to be a growing demand for remote patient monitoring to create quality care outcomes, ease of delivery and cost savings. Technology has been claimed to be a catalyst for change (Miller et al. 2009) and we may soon experience that a greater share of clinic visits today will be replaced by sophisticated technology encounters (personal *e*Health ecosystems).

Although most of the applications available today for diabetes educators are supplied by their healthcare providers, there is much to be gained from contemporary systems and diabetes educators may utilise HIT to:

- Acquire health and patient information from trusted sources,
- Follow clinical indicators and health outcomes from diabetes registers,
- Network with peers for decision support,
- Track individuals with high risk,
- Monitor and interact with patients to support patient self-care, and
- Predict the individual need for follow-up visits and examinations (in the future).

Diabetes management tools

Electronic health records and shared care

Electronic health records (EHR) collect data from multiple sources and are used as the primary source of information at the point of care. Improved access to patient-specific information provides benefits for the safety and quality of diabetes care. A more comprehensive description of EHR as a system of hardware, software, policies and processes may be found in the literature (Shortliffe and Perreault 2000). EHRs support patient care and facilitate communication between the diabetes care team. In addition to this comprehensive care, diabetes registries and diabetes care management systems assist in a more limited scope of diabetes care.

Healthcare has been radically decentralised (Giddens 2007) with distributed patient data repositories. One of the greatest challenges facing HIT today is the effective sharing of information among healthcare providers. Today's systems were designed primarily to facilitate administrative functions and a more open, standards-based HIT environment is required to capture, store, analyse and appropriately share information. Another barrier that needs to be amended is culture. Hospital care mirrors a knowledge-intensive service model with highly educated specialists and coordinated practice. These networks may be separated from primary care through organisational boundaries, but also to some degree by practice and identity that divide.

Resolutions to empower professionals in utilising HIT and to promote continuing development (Roberts 2009) have been set in motion (www. ukchip.org), but there are still restrictions to effective deployment, which is limited to connecting healthcare professionals and not patients. In the post-industrial society, we should be expecting empowered patients through a series of mechanisms, such as availability of information and personalisation of services and choice (Giddens 2007). HIT applications will emerge within a context of escalating citizens' use of technologies.

Diabetes registers

Disease registers are databases that contain condition-specific information for a group of patients and may generate patient reports or aggregate information across the population. Registers can be simple databases that require manual data entry or integrated registers where the database is updated by data retrieval from EHRs or other patient information systems. Integrated registers track all patient cases with a given disease or health condition in the population. In addition, some disease registers are based on administrative register data.

Registers are most often used for monitoring disease status at a population level and to track progress of the disease using process and outcome measures. Action plans may be based on these results in order to slow down the disease progress (Calvert et al. 2009). Integrated registers also provide feedback to providers of care on overall performance by patient and by population. IT-enabled diabetes management has the potential to improve care processes, delay diabetes complications and save costs (Bu et al. 2007). Consequently, diabetes registers have been created for various purposes (Huen et al. 2000; Gudbjörnsdottir et al. 2003; Gorus et al. 2004; Carstensen et al. 2008).

In Scotland at Tayside (DARTS), one of the first diabetes registers was created on the recommendation of NHS that regional diabetes registers should be established in the UK to facilitate systematic, population-based monitoring of outcomes of diabetes and to ensure that diabetes care is effective, efficient and equitable (Morris et al. 1997). A national systematic approach since 2000 towards quality improvement of diabetes care included the creation of managed clinical networks and the Scottish Diabetes Survey reporting annual improvements in diabetes care (Morris 2006). This has led to a significant change in clinical practice providing a national platform to underpin clinical networks of diabetes care.

There are variations in inclusion criteria of the registers as well as in the clinical registration of patients into the health information systems (Rollason et al. 2009). Such issues are important for the quality of the register, and it is important to analyse the completeness of registration in the diabetes registers. By applying four criteria to identify diabetes patients from two metropolitan cities in Finland, we extracted from 2008 EHR data over 37 600 diabetic patients giving a diabetes prevalence of 4.6% (Harno et al. 2010). These data were applied to track metrics of the care process and service use in the diabetic population.

Analytic tools

In designing an IT-enabled chronic disease management programme, there is a wide array of options (Adler-Milstein and Linden 2009). Besides provider tools for diabetes care, some are designed for identifying and stratifying the population at risk. The predictive modelling software is an analytic tool that stratifies a population according to medical need and risk. The sophisticated predictive models rely on multiple regression and artificial intelligence to inform predictions. A predictive model that is able to draw on medical, pharmacy and lab data as well as clinical data is better positioned to make more accurate predictions. Predictive models support the stratification process and predict the members of a chronically ill population who are most likely to incur high medical service utilisation in the near future. They enable a programme to intervene and avoid associated costs.

Personal assessment tools, such as health risk assessments, are survey-based instruments that assess health history and current health factors to determine health status and risk. These tools are available online for individuals (http://star.duodecim.fi/star/healthcheck.do) or they can be applied to all adults without a diagnosis during primary care visits (Department of Health 2008). Health checks have been utilised also on data recorded in EHRs, but since the data contain little information on lifestyle factors (physical activity and diet) computer templates will be needed to allow capture. These tools typically include psychometrically validated questions (e.g. behavioural, clinical) and more sophisticated versions rely on branching logic and delivering automated feedback based on responses.

Personal health tools and self-care

We may foresee people with diabetes who that are supported by personal health tools that engineer awareness and motivation and augment patients' power to take decisions and be proactive in taking responsibility for their health (Figure 12.2). The present tools, although less sophisticated, nevertheless help in guiding diabetics interactively to manage their health.

Disease management

- Remote patient monitoring
  - Weight
  - Blood pressure
  - Glucose
  - Temperature
  - Spirometer data
- Wireless network

Aging independently

- Medication compliance
- Assisted daily living
  - Bed pressure (sleep)
  - Bathroom sensor
  - Gas/water sensor
  - Emergency sensor

Health and wellness

- Weight loss
- Fitness
- "Worried well"
  - Weight
  - Blood pressure
  - Glucose
  - Cholesterol
  - Activity level
- Personal health records

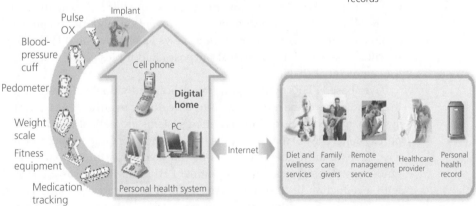

Figure 12.2 **The Continua Alliance has designed the guidelines towards the establishment of a personal eHealth ecosystem. These guidelines address the technical barriers and interoperability amongst different vendors allowing the transfer of data from self-management tools in this ecosystem. The diabetics that are supported by personal health tools engineer awareness and motivation, augment patients' power to take decisions and be proactive in taking responsibility for their health (www.continualliance.org).**

Personal health records and decision support systems

The personal health record (PHR) is the technical tool that will enable healthcare consumers to manage their health and their health-related behaviours in the twenty-first century. The PHR is a universally accessible, layperson comprehensible lifelong tool for managing relevant health information, promoting health maintenance and assisting with chronic disease management via an interactive, common data set of electronic health information and *e*Health tools.

Primary PHR functions fall into four general categories, based on use of information from the patient's perspective (Kaelber et al. 2008):

1. Information collection—PHR functions that help patients to enter their own health information and to retrieve their information from external sources.
2. Information sharing—PHR functions that allow patients to engage in one-way sharing of their health information with others.
3. Information exchange—PHR functions that allow patients to engage in two-way exchange with others.
4. Information self-management—PHR functions that allow patients to better manage their own health/healthcare.

Most previous PHR research is focused on the areas of information exchange and self-management, which includes patient-oriented disease information and decision support. Decision support systems (DSS) refer broadly to providing clinical knowledge and patient-related information, presented at appropriate times to enhance patient care (Jenders et al. 2007). DSS has been shown to increase quality and patient safety, improve adherence to guidelines for prevention and treatment, and avoid medication errors. Systematic reviews have shown that DSS can be useful across a variety of clinical purposes and topics (Garg et al. 2005; Kawamoto et al. 2005).

Payer-based PHRs apply algorithms to scan individual's claim data and then send alerts to the individual if they are due or overdue for a test. Such systems, termed 'sentinel' intervention systems are patient decision support systems (PDSS) that use clinical information contained in administrative claims data to identify errors in care and departures from clinical guidelines. The application of a sentinel PHR with PDSS was associated with a reduction in hospitalisation, medical costs and morbidity (Javitt et al. 2005). With health maintenance reminders, women were significantly more likely to receive PAP smears, but no difference was seen for the other reminders (Wright et al. 2008).

The sentinel systems need to be distinguished from point-of-care decision support, where information is derived from monitoring patient information. The use of online PHR linked to the EHR increased rates of diabetes-related medication adjustments, however no differences could be demonstrated between glycemic levels or risk factor control between the study arms after 1 year (Grant et al. 2008). Low rates of online patient registration and good baseline control among participants limited the intervention's impact on overall risk factor control. Another explanation may be that DSS reminders were not offered to patients, but to clinicians. Since provider-centric EHRs with DSS have had only modest impact on improving outcomes and results remain inconsistent, tethered PHRs and PDSS have been provided directly to patients.

Self-management tools and remote monitoring

Chronic disease is particularly suitable for remote management, especially when there is continuity between the patient and the care provider. Self-management tools (SMT) are used by patients and seek to improve chronic disease status by supporting patient self-care and encouraging appropriate utilisation of medical resources. Two primary subcategories of SMTs include (1) educational tools to educate users and (2) tools that enable patients to capture and review physiologic data. SMTs typically support a patient-focused intervention. Conceptually there are different roles that a patient can take in their self-management and these are reflected in the types of SMTs offered.

The California Health Foundation has proposed a framework in which self-management technologies support four patient roles:

1. Subordinate when technologies provide modest patient discretion within a strong supervisory context.
2. Structured when technologies involve more active but limited patient participation.
3. Collaborative when technologies involve patients using their own knowledge and making decisions jointly with clinicians.
4. Autonomous when technologies help patients take health matters in hand without major participation by clinicians. Most SMTs in diabetes fall into collaborative or autonomous categories.

During routine visits for most chronic diseases, monitoring to check on the progress or regress of the disease is performed by healthcare professionals. This requires individuals to choose what to monitor, when to monitor and how to adjust treatment. It can be done by nurse educators, patients or both. For patients, monitoring may provide a signal for action or motivation to adhere to treatment. The objective and methods of monitoring may change over the course of the treatment.

The course of monitoring has been divided into five phases (Glaszion et al. 2005). Achieving the desired target range and checking the individual's response to treatment are just some of the objectives of a drug titration phase or follow-up on wellness activities. During the maintenance phase, FTF visits may be extended when this is supplemented by patients' self-monitoring. Personalising treatment usually indicates some pragmatic trial and error. In case a shift from control has occurred, re-establishment of control often warrants shorter measurement intervals.

Thus, self-monitoring may have an impact through several means, including better selection of treatments based on individual response, better titration of treatment and patients' learning about non-treatment factors that alter control. The optimal process is not straightforward and a good monitoring strategy is needed: the choice of measurement(s), the choice of target range and the choice of measurement interval.

Remote monitoring enables providers to obtain symptom and physiologic data between visits. More advanced remote-monitoring solutions upload data directly from blood glucose meters, scales, blood pressure cuffs and other remote devices via phone lines or the Web. As opposed to self-management tools that capture physiologic data for patient use, remote monitoring may trigger an alert to health providers who can respond.

Systematic reviews of the literature have been conducted to illuminate the application of IT-enabling self-management with healthcare provider support (Solomon 2008) and the outcomes associated with SMT (Pare et al. 2007). Changes in patient adherence and levels of knowledge demonstrated significant improvements in both areas, but limitations in study design have led to inconclusive results. Although effects on patients' conditions remain inconclusive, SMTs produce accurate and reliable data, empower patients and improve their attitudes and behaviours. Regardless of nationality, socioeconomic status or age, patients comply with SMTs. The effects on clinical effectiveness outcomes e.g. decrease in the emergency visits, hospital admissions are more consistent in pulmonary and cardiac studies than diabetes and hypertension.

More recent randomised controlled trials in type 2 diabetics applying remote monitoring achieve significant improvements in glycosylated haemoglobin (Cho et al. 2006; Kim and Kim 2008; Quinn et al. 2008; Yoon and Kim 2008), but not in type 1 diabetics (Farmer et al. 2005). Despite these promising results, there is still some controversy on the use of SMTs. For example self-monitoring of blood glucose (SMBG) is seen as an essential part of type 1 diabetes treatment, but there exist dissenting opinions on its efficacy and cost-effectiveness in type 2 diabetes (Tatara et al. 2009).

The patients have several technical options for reporting measurement data. A recent study identified a total of 28 studies that examined mobile terminal-based applications or services to support self-management of diabetes (Gulliford 2008). Out of the 28 studies 20 used a mobile phone, but only a few of these are controlled studies. Only during the recent years has the usability of mobile applications become sufficient for such applications. In 10–15 years, remote monitoring may be accomplished with implantable measuring devices.

Internet service applications for remote monitoring are available from several sites e.g. bodybugg, BodyTrace, DirectLife, Fitbit, LoseIt and Withings. Once physiologic data is entered from scales, blood pressure cuffs or glucose monitors, SMTs may provide automatic feedback or direct the patients to relevant educational modules. Closely associated with SMTs are personal health records (PHR), which may operate as a repository of patient-entered data. PHRs may incorporate applications or modules that track trends over time or provide automatic feedback on physiologic data in the form of PDSS.

Summary

Chronic disease management is beginning to develop its own identity as an important component of healthcare. The awareness that uniform strategies can be equally effective than single interventions have underpinned the evolvement of systemic chronic care models where information technology plays a critical role in supporting these systems. Healthcare professionals make use of HIT to improve quality, safety and efficiency of care. Additional educational resources may be found in a recent clinical review (McLean et al. 2011) and supplementary knowledge on data communications has appeared in book form (Fong et al. 2011).

Reflective questions

Reflection is a key part of the person with diabetes' journey: it is equally important for health professionals to reflect on their journey as a health professional and educator. Following are some questions you might like to reflect on. It sometimes helps if you think about a person with diabetes you educated recently and felt you did not do the job as well as you would like to.

- Networks of practices supported by HIT enable care integration of diabetes patients. As diabetes educator in your region, how do you envision coordinating care using HIT?
- Patient-focused care means that healthcare is organised to maximise the effectiveness of patients to manage their chronic illness themselves. How may HIT be applied so that the patient becomes an active producer of health and not simply a passive recipient?
- Self-management tools allow diabetes educators remotely to address individual patient needs. In what ways could this opportunity improve the quality and safety of diabetes care?

References

Adler-Milstein, J., Linden, A. (2009). The use and evaluation of IT in chronic disease management. In: *Handbook of Research on Information Technology Management and Clinical Data Administration in Healthcare*. Vol. 1, ed. A. Dwiwedi, pp. 1–18. Medical Information Science Reference, Hershey, NY.

Berners-Lee, T. (2000). *Weaving the Web*. Texere Publishing Limited, London.

Brown, J.S., Duguid, P. (2002). *The Social Life of Information*. Harvard Business School Press, Boston, MA.

Bu, D., Pan, E., Walker, J. et al. (2007). Benefits of information technology-enabled diabetes management. *Diabetes Care* 30:1137–1142.

Calvert, M.J., Shankar, A., McManus, R.J., Lester, H., Freemantle, N. (2009). Effect of the quality and outcomes framework on diabetes care in the United Kingdom: Retrospective cohort study. *British Medical Journal* 338:1366–1370.

Campbell, R., Starkey, F., Holliday, J. et al. (2008). An informal school-based peer-led intervention for smoking prevention in adolescence (ASSIST): A cluster randomized trial. *Lancet* 371:1595–1602.

Carstensen, B., Kristensen, J.K., Ottosen, P., Borch-Johnsen, K. (2008). Steering Group of the National Diabetes Register. The Danish National Diabetes Register: trends in incidence, prevalence and mortality. *Diabetologia* 51(12):2187–2196.

Cho, J.-H., Chang, S., Kwon, H. et al. (2006). Long-term effects of the internet-based glucose monitoring system on HbA1c reduction and glucose stability: A 30-month follow-up study for diabetes management with a ubiquitous medical care system. *Diabetes Care* 29:2625–2631.

Department of Health. (2008). Putting prevention first-vascular checks: Risk assessment and management. www.dh.gov.uk

Eysenbach, G., Powell, J., Englesakis, M. et al. (2004). Health related virtual communities and electronic support groups: Systematic review of the effects of online peer to peer interactions. *British Medical Journal* 328(7449):1166. doi: 10.1136/bmj.328.7449.1166.

Farmer, A.J., Gibson, O.J., Dudley, C. et al. (2005). A randomized controlled trial of the effect of real-time telemedicine support on glycemic control in young adults with type 1 diabetes. *Diabetes Care* 28:2697–2702.

Fong, B., Fong, A.C.M., Li, C.K. (2011). *Telemedicine Technologies. Information Technologies in Mediicine and Telehealth*. John Wiley & Sons, Ltd., West Sussex.

Foster, G., Taylor, S.J.C., Eldridge, S., Ramsay, J., Griffiths, C.J. (2007). Self-management education programmes by lay leaders for people with chronic conditions. *Cochrane Database of Systematic Reviews* 17(4):CD005108. DOI: 10.1002/14651858.CD005108.pub2

Garg, A.X., Adhikari, N.K., McDonald, H. et al. (2005). Effects of computerized clinical decision support systems on practitioner performance and patient outcomes: A systematic review. *JAMA* 293:1261–1263.

Giddens, A. (2007). *Europe in the Global Age*. Polity Press, Cambridge.

Glaszion, P., Irwig, L., Mant, D. (2005). Monitoring in chronic disease: A rational approach. *British Medical Journal* 330:644–648.

Gorus, F.K., Weets, I., Couck, P., Pipeleers, D.G. (2004). Belgian Diabetes Registry. Epidemiology of type 1 and type 2 diabetes. The added value of diabetes registries for conducting clinical studies: the Belgian paradigm. *Acta Clinca Belgica* 59:1–13.

Grant, R.W., Wald, J.S., Schnipper, J.L. et al. (2008). Practice-linked online personal health records for type 2 diabetes mellitus. *Archives of Internal Medicine* 168:1776–1782.

Grusser Monika. (2011) Diabetes education for people with type 2—A European perspective. *Diabetes Voice* 56:34–37.

Gudbjörnsdottir, S., Cederholm, J., Nilsson, P.M., Eliasson, B., Steering Committee of the Swedish National Diabetes Register. (2003). The National Diabetes Register in Sweden: An implementation of the St. Vincent Declaration for Quality Improvement in Diabetes Care. *Diabetes Care* 26(4):1270–1276.

Gulliford, M. (2008). Self monitoring of blood glucose in type 2 diabetes. *British Medical Journal* 336:1139–1140.

Harno, K., Tolppanen, E.-M., Ranta, S., Suominen, L. (2010). An integrated regional register in care management. *Journal of the Finnish Medical Association* 65:2393–2398.

Holman, H., Lorig, K. (2000). Patients as partners in managing chronic disease. *British Medical Journal* 320:526–527.

Huen, K.F., Low, L.C., Wong, G.W. et al. (2000). Epidemiology of diabetes mellitus in children in Hong Kong: The Hong Kong childhood diabetes register. *Journal of Pediatric Endocrinology & Metabolism* 13(3):297–302.

Javitt, J.C., Steinberg, G., Locke, T. et al. (2005). Using a claims data-based sentinel system to improve compliance with clinical guidelines: Results of a randomized prospective study. *American Journal of Managed Care* 11(2):93–102.

Jenders, R.A., Osheroff, J.A., Sittig, D.F. et al. (2007). Recommendations for clinical decision support deployment: Synthesis of a roundtable of medical directors of information systems. *AMIA Annual Symposium Proceedings* 2007:359–363.

Kaelber, D.C., Jha, A.K., Johnston, D., Middleton, B., Bates, D.W. (2008). A research agenda for personal health records (PHRs). *Journal of the American Medical Informatics Association* 15:729–736.

Kawamoto, K., Houlihan, C.A., Balas, E.A., Lobach, D.A. (2005). Improving clinical practice using clinical decision support systems: A systematic review of trials to identify features critical to success. *British Medical Journal* 330:765–768.

Kim, S., Kim, H. (2008). Effectiveness of mobile and internet intervention in patients with obese type 2 diabetes. *International Journal of Medical Informatics* 77:399–404.

McLean, S., Protti, D., Sheikh, A. (2011). Telehealthcare for long term conditions. *British Medical Journal* 342:374–378.

Mezrich, B. (2010) *The Accidental Billionaires: The Founding of Facebook, a Tale of Sex, Money, Genius and Betrayal*. Anchor Books, New York.

Miller, H.D., Yasnoff, W.A., Burde, H.A. (2009) *Personal Health Records. The Essential Missing Element in 21st Century Healthcare*. HIMSS, Chicago, IL.

Morris, A. (2006). Outcomes from a national diabetes IT network: The Scottish experience. *Diabetic Medicine* 23(suppl 4):1208.

Morris, A.D., Boyle, D.I.R., MacAlpine, R. et al. (1997). The diabetes audit and research in Tayside Scotland (darts) study: Electronic linkage to create a diabetes register. *British Medical Journal* 315:524–528.

Mulcahy, K., Maryniuk, M., Peeples, M. et al. (2003). Diabetes self-management education core outcomes measures. *The Diabetes Educator* 29:768–803.

Murray, E. (2008a). Providing information for patients is insufficient on its own to improve clinical outcomes. *British Medical Journal* 337:306–307.

Murray, E. (2008b). Internet-delivered treatments for long-term conditions: Strategies, efficiency and cost-effectiveness. *Expert Review of Pharmaco-economics & Outcomes Research* 8:261–272.

O'Connor, A.M., Stacey, D., Legare, F. (2008). Coaching to support patients in making decisions. *British Medical Journal* 336:228–229.

Pare, G., Mirou, J., Sicotte, C. (2007). Systematic review of home telemonitoring for chronic diseases: The evidence base. *JAMIA* 14:269–277.

Quinn, C.C., Clough, S.S., Minor, J.M., Lender, D., Okafor, M.C., Gruber-Baldini, A. (2008). WellDoc mobile diabetes management randomized controlled trial: Change in clinical and behavioral outcomes and patient and physician satisfaction. *Diabetes Technology & Therapeutics* 10:160–168.

Roberts, J.M. (2009). Current challenges in empowering clinicians to utilize technology. In *Handbook of Research on Information Technology Management and Clinical Data Administration in Healthcare*. ed. A. Dwivedi, pp. 507–520. Medical Information Science Reference, Hershey, NY.

Rollason, W., Khunti, K., de Lusignan, S. (2009). Variation in the recording of diabetes diagnostic data in primary care computer systems: Implications for the quality of care. *Informatics in Primary Care* 17(2):113–119.

Rubak, S., Sandbeak, A., Lauritzen, T., Christensen, B. (2005). Motivational interviewing: A systematic review and meta-analysis. *British Journal of General Practice* 55:305–312.

Shortliffe, E.H., Perreault, L.E., eds. (2000). *Medical Informatics*. Springer-Verlag, New York, Berlin, Heidelberg.

Solomon, M.R. (2008). Information technology to support self-management in chronic care. A systematic review. *Dis Manage Health Outcomes* 16:391–401.

Tatara, N., Årsand, E., Nilsen, H., Hartvigsen, G. (2009). A review of mobile terminal-based applications for self-management of patients with diabetes. *International Conference on eHealth, Telemedicine and Social Medicine (eTELEMED 2009)*. Cancun, p. 14.

Wright, A., Poon, E.G., Wald, J. et al. (November 2008). Effectiveness of health maintenance reminders provided directly to patients. *AMIA Annual Symposium Proceedings* 6:1183.

Yoon, K., Kim, H. (2008). A short message service by cellular phone in type 2 diabetic patients for 12 months. *International Journal of Medical Informatics* 79:256–261.

13 Leadership—Know Yourself: Influence Others

Trisha Dunning AM

Deakin University and Barwon Health, Geelong, Victoria, Australia

Not the cry, but the flight of a wild duck, leads the flock to fly and follow.
(Chinese Proverb)

Introduction

When I was being interviewed for my current job, a very high-ranking senior academic on the interview panel asked:

How would you recognise a leader, if you saw one walking along the waterfront?

I did *not* expect that question, and had not prepared for it. The names and traits of some my favourite leaders chased each other through my mind. I glanced out the window at the waterfront. I could not see *any* leaders walking along it, but there was a scuttle of children laughing and playing

I almost said, *The Pied Piper: I would know him anywhere by his music and the rats following him.*

But this was a serious interview! I could not discuss the Pied Piper, King Arthur, Julius Caesar or Eleanor of Aquitaine—I was sure he meant a more modern leader. So I described some of the traits I admired in these leaders. Thankfully, he nodded thoughtfully then said:

*Now describe **your** leadership style.*

I found the question challenging, but later I reflected on my personal view and worldviews about leadership. Eventually, that academic's question became the impetus for this chapter.

Diabetes Education: Art, Science and Evidence, First Edition. Edited by Trisha Dunning AM.
© 2013 John Wiley & Sons, Ltd. Published 2013 by John Wiley & Sons, Ltd.

The purpose of Chapter 13 is to briefly explore leadership from a historical perspective, outline some of the definitions of leadership and the main leadership theories and styles, and the core and advanced competencies leaders require to lead effectively. However, the main focus of the chapter leadership is on leadership in diabetes education and care, given that leadership is a core component of the diabetes educator role.

Leadership: a brief historical perspective

Leadership is an intriguing concept. Many images of leaders have their roots in conflict where leadership was seen as outwitting opponents and taking control. There are five broad generations of leadership theories:

1. great man
2. trait
3. behaviour
4. contingency
5. transformational.

Leadership was a broad concept in the ancient world that suited the environment and context at the time. Most ancient leaders were men, but there were a few notable women who blazed their mark on history, for example Boudicca, Hatshepsut and Cleopatra, and more recently Florence Nightingale and Maggie Thatcher. Leadership became more complex as society and technology advanced.

In the 1900s, the focus was on the 'Great Man' theory. Leadership was regarded as the role of people from the privileged ranks of society or geniuses. 'Group theories' emerged in the 1930s during the Great Depression when psychologists in the United States were studying groups that had a democratic leadership style. They concluded, democratic leadership was possible and was more effective. Consequently, an egalitarian view of leadership evolved. Later research indicated that leadership behaviours in small groups is not necessarily transferable to large groups or organisations.

During World War II, people began to debate what traits leaders needed to win the war but no consensus was reached: and a comprehensive literature review indicated the evidence was contradictory (Stogdill 1948). Later, Stogdill and other researchers hypothesised about behavioural leadership styles, but were not able to determine which behaviours or behavioural patterns distinguished leaders.

Two distinct leadership behaviour categories were described: concern for tasks and concern for people (House and Aditya 1997). Some experts suggest 'the ultimate test of [leadership] should be how the leader's colleagues behave' (Zenger et al. 2009). However, many confounding factors are likely to influence followers' behaviour besides the leader. Therefore, making the leader totally accountable for followers' behaviour may be too simplistic.

Behaviour leadership theories were followed by transformational leadership theories in the 1970s. Transformational leaders communicate with and engage and mentor followers. Many experts believe transformational leadership is the ideal. Skill at effecting change emerged as an essential leadership trait in the 1990s (Yuki et al. 2002). Change-oriented behaviours include utilising and undertaking research to guide practice (Gifford et al. 2007).

Traditional healthcare leadership models were consistent with organisational theory and focused on influencing other people to accomplish organisational goals. Modern healthcare services/organisations are expected to be effective, competitive, high performing, cost-effective and safe. To achieve these high pressure stretch goals, the leaders must find ways to engage with and motivate staff, as well as being mindful of their own well-being. The latter is important for ethical reasons, as well as to ensure the organisation meets its goals.

Alimo-Metcalfe (2008) developed a leadership model, Engaging Leadership, which enables organisations to develop leaders and create an environment where staff can remain motivated, perform optimally and have less stress. Robinson et al. (2004) defined 'engagement' as:

A positive attitude held by the employee towards the organisation and its values. An engaged employee is aware of business context, and works with colleagues to improve performance within the job for the benefit of the organization.

Alimo-Metcalfe's (2008) Model of Engaging Leadership includes:

- Engaging with individuals
- Engaging the organisation
- Moving forward together by engaging stakeholders
- Personal qualities and values.

Research suggests organisations with a culture of engagement perform better than their competitors (Towers Perin 2005; Watson-Wyatt 2006). Leadership in high performing organisations:

- Engages key stakeholders
- Has a shared vision of 'a quality, safe service'
- Functions in collaborative, non-hierarchical teams
- Fosters a supportive culture
- Is an effective change agent (Alimo-Metcalfe 2008).

Thus, leadership styles slowly evolved from leader-follower-dyads to more collaborative leadership styles that include modern contingency models that focus on the context in which leaders operate (Reicher et al. 2007).

What is leadership and what/who is a leader?

There are many definitions of leadership. Many people still believe a leader is being the person out in front; an entrenched hangover from the Great Man theory. Some diabetes educator's experiences indicate Great Man leadership styles still exist and are a challenge or barrier to diabetes educators in some countries undertaking leadership roles. For example, one educator said:

Hierarchical [leadership] *models still exist, usually male medical dominated. They do not want to be challenged, to discuss things, they think their knowledge is greater and their position superior.*

Dunning and Manias (2008, pp. 392–398)

One could ask whether these male medical leaders' thinking is outdated. The Great Man leadership style is not fit for purpose in modern diabetes care where the 'gold standard' is held out to be interdisciplinary team care. Effective leaders set the direction and influence people to follow the direction. The way the leader sets the direction and influences people depends on a range of factors, most particularly their concept of leadership and leadership style. One definition of leadership states:

Leadership means the ability to shape what followers actually want to do, not the act of enforcing compliance using rewards and punishments.

Reicher et al. (2007)

Encouraging followers to 'want to do' is an art. It is impossible without the cooperation of and support from followers. The term 'follower' is interesting, and could be a hangover from the Great Man theory. I have used it in this chapter for expediency, but it does not accord with group or transformational leadership theories, or with consumer engagement and person-centred holistic care.

Encouraging followers is a multidimensional process that includes behaviours, attitudes and skills applied to the context, in this case diabetes education and care, including educating individuals and self. Thus, although leadership traits are important, leaders must position themselves within the group and be clearly representative of the group to be credible. Some leadership styles and the key leader traits of the styles are shown in Table 13.1.

Table 13.1   **Common leadership styles (Bielby Consulting 2012).**

Leadership style	Main features of the style, key traits of leaders who use the style
Directive	• Have firm views about how and when things should be done • Dislikes followers showing independent thinking or initiative • Goal orientated and concerned with the results • Monitors followers' performance • Rarely invites others to contribute ideas
Delegative	• Delegates work to followers • Process of delegation may or may not involve consulting with followers, i.e. assigns work rather than seeks active input into how it could be accomplished • Once work is delegated provides little supervision, support
Participative	• Concerned with optimal team performance • Values group discussion and consensus • Likes to give each follower the opportunity to express their point of view • Unlikely to impose own point of view or opinions on followers • Democratic
Consultative	• Combines elements of democratic and directive leadership styles • Values group discussion but tends to encourage individuals to contribute • Usually makes the final decision • Effectiveness depends on the individuals' capacity to consider the advantages and disadvantages and to persuade followers to accept their decision
Negotiative	• Uses incentives to encourage followers to work towards objectives and work in a particular way • Relies on their ability to persuade followers to achieve objectives • Have well-developed management skills, which they use to modify their style to suit particular circumstances • Strong desire to achieve so sometimes uses unconventional ways to achieve the objectives
Followers' styles	**Key traits of followers who adopt the style**
Receptive-subordinate	• Accommodating • Wants to complete work assigned to them on time • Rarely suggests innovative ideas
Self-reliant subordinate	• Likes to share their ideas • Has innovative, imaginative ideas • Concerned with achieving results
Collaborative subordinate	• Believes team problem-solving capacity is greater than the capacity of individuals • Concerned that the *team* achieves its objectives • Enjoys group discussions • Has and shares innovative ideas but is prepared to discuss other people's ideas • Believes in and accepts constructive criticism but is uncomfortable about discussing other people's weaknesses

(Continued)

Table 13.1   (*continued*)

Informative subordinate	• Has well thought out ideas
	• Generates creative ideas and solutions to problems
	• Capable of detailed critical analysis of their own and other people's ideas and work
Reciprocating subordinate	• Rarely phased by criticism or problems when things do not go as per plan
	• Happy to promote their own ideas or to discuss and negotiate with others
	• Holds string views

However, different researchers and authors use many different terms to describe leadership styles, for example, autocratic, democratic, servant, laissez-fair, adaptive, appreciative, authentic, charismatic, dynamic, heroic and situational, but most are encompassed in the styles described. The second part of the table outlines the various styles followers adopt.

Leader functions

Leading is different from managing but there are many similarities, and both encompass four major functions:

1. Planning and setting relevant clear, measurable and achievable and agreed objectives.
2. Organising work, resources and staff to ensure the work is completed and goals achieved.
3. Monitoring/evaluating outcomes, targets, indicators or impacts, depending on the objective.
4. Communicating and disseminating relevant information to relevant stakeholders.

Leaders need to maintain a balance between leading and managing and be able to use different skills and styles at different times to suit the circumstance or situation.

Leadership philosophies, theories and models

The terms 'philosophy', 'theory' and 'model' are often used interchangeably. Generally, a philosophy is a broad set of beliefs derived from long observation and/or research. A theory refers to an idea or hunch about why 'something' happens, based on observations, research and philosophies. Theories are used to explain the traits needed to be effective leaders (Table 13.2). In contrast, a model describes a theory of leadership that includes the core and extended role components and leadership attribute. A key component of leadership philosophies, theories and models is leadership styles.

Table 13.2   **Some key traits effective leaders need: although common desirable traits are described in the literature, the most desirable trait depends on the group being led and the context leadership occurs in.**

- Has a vision that is clearly articulated and communicated to followers
- Has values congruent with and understands the values and opinions of followers/colleagues
- Behaves ethically and responsibly
- Effectively communicates ideas and listens to comments and ideas from followers
- Is able to fit seamlessly into the group when a shared social identity exists as is the case with diabetes education. Such a leader must belong to the group and exemplify the factors that make the group different from other groups
- Is fair and non-judgemental
- Solves problems and makes decisions
- Is creative, innovative and flexible
- Is capable of planning, delegating, directing, counselling and mentoring colleagues and facilitating meetings
- Is forward thinking and able to 'see the trees *and* the wood', i.e. details as well as the big picture

In order to competently lead others, the individual must be able to lead themselves.

Leadership styles

Leadership style refers to how an individual acts in their leadership capacity. Researchers/theorists have identified several main styles, but they use various terms to describe each style. Table 13.1 outlines commonly used descriptors applied to leadership styles as well as follower styles (Beilby Consulting 2012). Importantly, there is no right style, but adaptability and flexibility are important personal leader attributes.

The leadership style most likely to be effective depends on:

- The prevailing situation and context
- The people the leader works with
- The leader's personal characteristics.

A leadership qualities checklist and a leadership questionnaire that can help people identify their personal leadership characteristics can be accessed on http://www.teamtechnology.co.uk/leadership-qualities.html

Leadership competencies and attributes

Diabetes health professionals (HPs) are very familiar with competencies and some diabetes education associations describe core leadership and management competencies (Australian Diabetes Educators Association (ADEA) 2008). However, most apply to management. The competencies needed to lead in successively more complex situations, from individuals to groups, to organisations and beyond, become successively more complex. These ADEA core competencies describe the minimum needed to lead others rather than the extended domain competencies needed in

Table 13.3   **Competencies a leader requires to function effectively.**

Leading others	Leading self
Cares for own health and wellness	Cares for own health and wellness
Ability to make decisions	Able to reflect to develop self- and professional knowledge
Effective communication skills, in particular listening	Committed to continuing professional development
Plans	Respects themselves
Sets goals	Honest with self
Problem solving	Able to solve problems
Behaves ethically, e.g. respects individuals	
Social responsibility	
Creative and innovative	
Uses systems thinking and takes a broad view and identify patterns, trends and processes	
Able to resolve conflict	
Able to reflect to develop self- and professional knowledge	
Productive	

Competencies are usually acquired in a cumulative fashion through opportunity, mentoring, role modelling and experience. Core competencies refer to the minimum competencies needed to lead others. It is essential competence is maintained in all domains.

some leadership roles. The latter include managing 'power and influence', political awareness and managing organisational change.

Whether the leader is leading a team or group, or working with an individual they need a core set of knowledge and competence to function effectively. In addition, they have other attributes that enhance their effectiveness. Importantly, a leader cannot effectively lead other people if they cannot lead themselves. Significantly, the competencies and attributes needed to lead in one situation might not automatically apply in other situations or contexts. The core leadership competencies are shown in Table 13.3 and can be surmised from the following:

The play *The Admirable Crichton* Barrie (1902) illustrates the particular leadership competencies required in two quite different situations, very clearly. Briefly, Lord Loam and his butler Crichton live by and believe in the class system. In fact Crichton says: '*it is a natural outcome of civilised society*'. Lord Loam, his family, friends and Crichton become shipwrecked on a deserted tropical island. Crichton is the only person in the group with the skills needed to survive in this very different environment. Crichton reluctantly assumes the leadership role and becomes more competent as a leader as he becomes more experienced and is finally accepted as the leader by his social superiors, and referred to as 'Guv'.

The film *Twelve O'clock High* Bartlett et al. (1949) is set during the World War II when a squadron begins to suffer heavy losses and morale declines.

The Squadron Leader, who has a people-oriented leadership style, is replaced by a dictatorial leader who restores the squadron's pride and reduces losses. *Twelve O'clock High* shows dictatorial leadership styles might be appropriate in some situations. Interestingly, Hitler, one of history's most despised dictators, was only able to rise to power because of the situation in Germany after World War I and the demoralising conditions the Germans found themselves in after the Treaty of Versailles, as well as the apathy of other world leaders.

von Goethe (1751–1858) wrote a very insightful description of leadership that involved self-reflection. He said:

> *I have come to the frightening conclusion that I am the decisive element.*
> *It is my personal approach that creates the climate.*
> *It is my daily mood that makes the weather.*
> *I possess tremendous power to make life miserable or joyous.*
> *I can be a tool of torture or an instrument of inspiration.*
> *I can humiliate humor or heal.*

One could assume from von Goethe's self-observation that the ultimate test of an effective leader might be how their followers behave, as Zenger et al. (2009 p. 9) suggested. However, there are many confounding variables that would need to be accounted for. Thus, followers' behaviour may only be a surrogate marker of the leader's effectiveness. We can apply the same thinking to diabetes education and management outcomes where we base the effectiveness of HPs' recommendation on the person with diabetes' metabolic and other self-care outcomes. People with diabetes' outcomes are also subject to many confounders and some are probably also only surrogate markers of diabetes educator/education effectiveness.

There is a variety of valid tools to measure these parameters, *but* how often do HPs measure their own performance and its effect on the people with diabetes' outcomes? Diabetes educators need to consider measuring their own performance as rigorously as they measure that of people with diabetes using more useful tools than 'patient satisfaction surveys' and quality of teaching scores, both of which are flawed. We could consider measuring the educator's ability to establish and maintain a therapeutic relationship (Dunning 2011). Self-reflection is essential to leadership and is part of continuing professional development (CPD). Reflection could be a good starting point: in fact it is a required component of the recently revised ADEA CPD process.

As indicated, von Goethe's comment highlights the importance and power of self-reflection. Self-reflection is not easy, but it is critical to self-improvement in any role. Reflection does not refer to 'self-talk' that goes on in most people's head a lot of the time. Self-reflection is a constructive, purposeful introspective process undertaken to learn more about one's nature, purpose and performance. It is essential to an individual's personal and professional development. It also demonstrates a leader's security and authenticity. von Goethe's words show leaders create an atmosphere (climate) that can inspire or motivate or wound and demotivate. Building follower's self-efficacy and reflective ability is more likely to motivate. Importantly, building other people's self-efficacy builds the leader's self-efficacy.

Leadership education and care of people with diabetes

Leadership is essential in all aspects of diabetes education and care: service planning and development, clinical care, including individual consultations, and research. Mullins (2009) described leadership as a relationship where one person influences and changes another. The type of influence the leader exerts depends on their leadership style and the quality of the relationship (see Chapter 3). Ideally, leaders and followers (educators and people with diabetes) influence each other and cogenerate information. Both parties must adapt to accommodate each other's points of view. If mutual adaptation does not occur, the encounter may not be as effective as it could have been.

The core components of the diabetes educator role are clinical care, education, research and leadership: leadership is inherent in all components. Some ways diabetes educators demonstrate leadership is through:

- Developing local, national and international policies, guidelines and service models.
- Advocating for people with diabetes, the profession and the way of working, e.g. empowerment models and chronic disease models.
- Providing clinical governance.
- Providing expert clinical care and education.
- Mentoring colleagues.
- Working on committees.
- Undertaking and promulgating research to generate and support the evidence base of the profession. Opinion leaders such as diabetes educators can promote changes (Flodgren et al. 2011), but the effectiveness varies among studies. Many factors could account for the variability including methodological differences but leadership style could also play a role.

There are many outstanding diabetes educator leaders, and many more are emerging. However, the profession rarely proactively identifies and mentors future leaders to develop a critical mass of positive educator leaders, although clinical mentoring does occur within teams. Once a leader emerges that individual often seeks informal and formal mentors, but leader identification, succession planning and sustainability, rarely, if ever, occurs nationally or internationally. Yet diabetes educators are able to identify their leaders and the attributes they value (Dunning and Manias 2008; Dunning 2012).

Leadership in diabetes clinical care

Diabetes clinical care is difficult to separate from education. Educators (and people with diabetes) expect their leaders (and leaders expect themselves) to be clinically competent (Dunning and Manias 2008). Leadership 'status' is often accorded by colleagues rather than conferred as a formal position title, unlike the titles diabetes education manager, diabetes nurse consultant, diabetes specialist, although leadership is inherent in these roles.

Transformational and group leadership theories appear to accord with diabetes clinical care and the philosophy of holistic person-centred care that actively involves people with diabetes in their care. In western countries, diabetes educators work in interdisciplinary teams, but many are also autonomous.

Leadership in diabetes education

Katzenmeyer and Moller (2009 p. 2) suggested the only way teacher quality will improve is if the teachers learn to teach better. The statement was made about school teachers in light of criticism about the quality of the teaching and poor student outcomes. Diabetes educators also need to consider the hard reality that many people with diabetes do not achieve 'optimal outcomes': 'targets' and 'good control'. Educators need to reflect, like von Goethe did, about whether some of the reason people with diabetes do not achieve optimal outcomes is due to ineffective teaching and clinical care. Granted, educators are expected to cope with increasing numbers of people with diabetes with fewer resources and personnel and fulfil other administrative requirements that compromise education time.

Significantly, diabetes educators regard clinical and education expertise as key leadership competencies (Dunning and Manias 2008; Dunning 2012), which is consistent with the literature (Table 13.4).

Leadership in diabetes research

As stated, research engagement in its broadest meaning (Dunning 2011) is the responsibility of all HPs including diabetes educators, yet many diabetes educators feel research should not be an essential CPD category.

Table 13.4 **Key leadership attributes and competencies that emerged from a survey of 60 Australian diabetes educators their colleagues regard as leaders and those that emerged in a survey of 10 international diabetes education leaders.**

Australian diabetes educator leaders	International diabetes education leaders
Has a high profile and is well connected	Willing to share
Passion	Has a high profile and is well connected
Clinical competence and credibility	Politically aware
Visionary	Commitment
Problem-solver	Passionate
Mentor	Clinical competence and credibility
Does not need to put self forward 'not always out in front'	Values science (research), publishes and is quoted by others
Excellent communication and listening skills	Visionary
Confident and articulate	Problem-solver
Has fun and is fun to be with	Ability to delegate
Works hard	Asks questions
Some are quiet achievers	Committed to self-development
Able to see the big picture	Mentors
	Takes risks
	Excellent communication and listening skills
	Open minded
	Optimistic
	Confident
	Praises when relevant
	Instils confidence
	Behaves ethically and responsibly
	Has fun and is fun to be with
	Works hard
	Change agent
	Does not need to put self forward 'not always out in front'
	Leads by example

These are not in any priority order or category.

This belief is mostly predicated on a narrow view of what research engagement means, but it is a major concern, given that all diabetes educators practise in a climate of evidence-based care and could be regarded as opinion leaders. Diabetes educator's research behaviours comprise two main categories: facilitative and regulatory.

Facilitative

- Engaging in and encouraging research and research utilisation
- Sharing research information through publications, journal clubs and conference presentations

- Integrating relevant research findings into guidelines and policies and in their own clinical care and education
- Explaining research findings to people with diabetes, their carers and colleagues (Dunning 2011).

Regulatory

- Complying with relevant regulatory requirements, codes of ethics, professional conduct and other practice standards.
- Monitoring their own performance, for example through reflection, and the annual CPD process
- Undertaking practice audits/evaluations and using the findings to improve care.

What do diabetes educators think about leadership?

Dunning and Manias (2008) explored the leadership perceptions of 60 Australian diabetes educators their peers regarded as diabetes education leaders. The responses of nominated educators indicated they also regarded themselves as leaders, primarily because they:

- Had worked as a diabetes educator for a long time
- Mentored colleagues
- Worked in a range of practice settings and thus acquired a range of skills and knowledge that broadened their experience, outlook and clinical skills
- Attended conferences and professional development forums
- Had a high profile.

These views reflected the views of the educators who nominated them. They were nominated because they had worked in the role a long time, mentored and supervised colleagues, had a high profile, worked in niche areas such as wound management and were clinically competent.

A thematic analysis of a range of books and papers on leadership revealed a long list of skills and attributes leaders need to be effective. These are not all used at the same time or in every situation, but need to be available when the situation/context arises. Sometimes, people are not aware they are leaders until a situation arises and they have to cope or survive—for example, leaders who emerge during disasters and conflicts: as Lao Tzu said *'When the time is right the master* [leader] *will appear'* (1999 translated by Mitchell).

Some key leadership attributes are shown in Table 13.4, which also shows the attributes and skills that emerged in Dunning and Manias' (2008) survey and in a survey of international diabetes educator leaders I conducted in 2011 to inform the content of this chapter cited as Dunning

> **Box 13.1   Questions used to explore 16 randomly selected international diabetes educators' perceptions of leadership in 2011**
>
> 1. How would you define a leader?
> 2. What are the key *attributes* of a leader in diabetes education and management?
> 3. What key *attitudes* do leaders in diabetes education and management have in common?
> 4. How do diabetes educator leaders develop their leadership skills?
> 5. Briefly outline how you became a leader in diabetes education and management.
> 6. What challenges do/did you face on your leadership journey?
> 7. What factors facilitated your journey?
> 8. What continues to inspire you to perform your leadership role?
> 9. Who do you consider to be an outstanding diabetes education leader?
> 10. What makes them an outstanding leader?
> 11. Briefly outline their leadership style.
> 12. Please make any other comments.

2012. I randomly selected and invited 16 outstanding diabetes educator leaders from around the world to complete an anonymous questionnaire that asked 12 open questions about leaders and leadership (see Box 13.1). I am very grateful to the ten who responded and who wrote so much.

How can we grow diabetes education leaders?

Leadership appears to develop naturally in groups and is often shared among the group. Have you ever watched a flock of wild geese flying? Have you thought about the vast distances these migratory birds fly and the toll on the lead bird? They take it in turns to fly lead bird, that way they conserve the energy of the group and increase its chances of survival. One could ask whether diabetes educators should take a turn flying lead bird. Certainly they should lead by example, as the quote at the beginning of the chapter describes.

Although diabetes educators can identify leaders and desirable leader attributes, one could ask whether there is an agreed definition of diabetes education leadership. Is such a definition possible?

A suggested draft definition of diabetes education leadership is as follows:

Diabetes education leaders are reflective experts who lead within and beyond clinical care and education. They identify with and contribute to society and to a community of diabetes educator learning, clinical excellence, research development and research utilisation. They are committed to continuing professional and personal development for themselves and their colleagues to help people with diabetes and their families/carers achieve the best possible self-care and outcomes. They take responsibility for their leadership decisions.

The International Diabetes Federation (IDF) D-net diabetes education network is an example of an international community of learning and is an ideal avenue for discussing leadership. Such discussion could also occur during the IDF World Congress Diabetes Educator Forum. In addition, diabetes educator training curricula could be revised to formally include leadership training and developing core leadership competencies. Extended competencies could be developed within a formal mentoring model, combined with some theoretical information that could be delivered as self-directed learning.

Individually, educators can participate in conferences and networks, build positive relationships and seek out mentors formally and informally to develop their philosophy of leadership, and become known and develop leadership knowledge and competence. Some diabetes educators indicate that they:

share company with the movers and groovers to develop my profile. It is important to be seen with the right people, even if it is bathing in reflected glory.

Dunning and Manias (2008)

Summary

The most important point about leadership is encapsulated in the Chinese proverb at the beginning of the chapter and in von Goethe's reflection. Effective leadership depends on the leader being adaptable and flexible, having excellent people skills and managing change. Diabetes educators appear to have a common understanding of what diabetes education leadership is, and respect leadership roles.

There is always capacity to do better. Thus, self-reflection is essential for all leaders and educators and interdisciplinary teams. Reflection helps develop self-awareness and confidence. As Adlai Stevenson said:

Believe in yourself. It's hard to lead a cavalry charge if you think you look funny on a horse.

But if you fall off the horse, reflect, then get back on and try again.

> **Reflective questions**
>
> Reflection is essential to learning. It is a key part of the person with diabetes' journey and it is equally important for HPs to reflect on their journey as carers and educators. The following statements or questions may help you reflect. It sometimes helps if you think about a recent encounter with a person with diabetes where you felt the encounter did not go as well as you would like.
>
> - Use the questionnaire in Box 13.1 to reflect on your views about leadership.
> - How do they compare with von Goethe's personal reflection on page 223?
> - Is the draft definition of diabetes education leadership congruent with your views about diabetes education leadership?
> - Consider the leader and follower styles outlined in Table 13.4. Which follower styles would work best with which leader styles?
>
> Since so much of this book concerns language and philosophy as well as science, it is fitting to end it with a Rubaiyat (stanza) from a book that accompanies me everywhere: *The Rubaiyat of Omar Khayyam*. Omar was praised for his proficiency in science and for his wisdom. The following Rubaiyat, number 28, attests to his proficiency as a philosopher and writer.
>
> *The Moving Finger writes; and having writ,*
> *Moves on: nor all thy Piety nor Wit*
> *Shall lure it back to cancel half a Line,*
> *Nor all thy Tears wash out a Word of it.*
> The Rubaiyat of Omar Khayyam (1953)

Acknowledgements

The following people responded to an anonymous questionnaire about leadership, which is referred to in the chapter: Michelle Robins, Adjunct Professor Margaret McGill AM, Dr Sheridan Waldron, Dr Bodil Rasmussen, Dr Martha Funnell, Dr Seyda Ozcan, Eva Kan, Anne Belton, Anne Marie Felton, Dr Linda Siminerio and Dr Ming Yeong Tan.

References

Alimo-Metcalfe B. (2008) Building leadership capacity through engaging leadership. Report of the 12th World Congress, London.

Australian Diabetes Educators Association (ADEA). (2008) *National Core Competencies for Credentialled Diabetes Educators*. Canberra, ADEA.

Barrie J. (1902) The Admirable Crichton. A stage play first performed on November 4th 1902. London, Duke of York Theatre.

Bartlett S, King H, Lay B. (1949) *Twelve O'Clock High*. A film by Twentieth Century Fox that premiered on the 21st December 1949. Los Angeles, CA.

Beilby Consulting. (2012) Leadership styles. http://www.beilby.com.au/index.php?id=84 (accessed July 2011).

Dunning T. (2011a) Research and diabetes nursing. Part 1, terms of engagement. *Journal of Diabetes Nursing* 15(1):9–14.

Dunning T (2011b) Chronic disease self-management: what do we measure? *Journal of Nursing and Health Care* 15(1):251–253.

Dunning T. (2012) International diabetes educators' leaders' perceptions of leadership. Unpublished survey undertaken as part of the research for this chapter.

Dunning T, Manias E. (2008) Diabetes nurse educators' perceptions of leadership characteristics. *Journal of Diabetes Nursing* 12(10):392–398.

Flodgren G, Parmelli E, Doumit G, O' Brien M, Grimshaw J, Eccles M. (2011) Local opinion leaders: Effects on professional practice and health outcomes. *Cochrane Database of Systematic Reviews* 10(8):CE000125. DOI:10.1002/14651858. CD000125.

Gifford W, Davies B, Edwards N, Griffin P, Lybanon V. (2007) Managerial leadership for nurses' use of research evidence: An integrative review of the literature. *World Views on Evidence-Based Nursing* 4(3):126–145.

von Goethe J. (1751–1858) Brian Johnson philosopher's notes self-development inspirational quotes. www.thelugeman.com/motivational-quotes.htm (accessed December 2011).

House R, Aditya R. (1997) The social scientific study of leadership: Quo Vadis? *Journal of Management* 23:409–473.

Katzenmeyer M, Moller G. (2009) *Awakening the Sleeping Giant: Helping Teachers Develop as Leaders*. California, Corwin, p. 9.

Lao Tzu (1999 translation) *Tao Te Ching: An Illustrated Journey* Translated by Mitchell S. London Francis Lincoln.

Mullins I. (2009) *Management and Organizational Behaviour* (8th edn.). Harlow, Financial Time Prentice Hall.

Reicher S, Haslam S, Platow M. (2007) The new psychology of leadership. *Scientific American Mind*. August/September:22–29.

Robinson D, Perrymon D, Hayday S. (2004) The drivers of employee engagement. Institute for Employment Studies, Report 406. Sussex.

Stogdill R. (1948) Personal factors associated with leadership: A survey of the literature. *Journal of Psychology* 25:35–71.

The Rubaiyat of Omar Khayyam. (1953) Translated by Edward Fitzgerald (first translation). London, Ward, Lock & Co.

Towers P. (2005) Reconnecting with Employees: Quantifying the Value of Engaging the Workforce. London.

Watson-Wyatt. (2006) *Effective Communication: A Leading Indicator of Financial Performance*. Report 2005/2006. Communication ROI Study.

Yuki G, Gordon A, Taber T. (2002) A hierarchical taxonomy of leadership behaviour: Integrating a half century of behaviour research. *Journal of Leadership and Organisational Studies* 19:15–32.

Zenger J, Folkman J, Edinger S. (2009) *The Inspiring Leader*. Chicago, McGraw Hill, p. 28.

Appendix

The appendix is a list of some novels, poetry, people's accounts of their illnesses and movies that portray human nature and the way people cope with life situations. They help explain people's behaviours, attitudes, explanatory models and stories. Many portray examples of teachers, learners, teaching and learning, good and not so good, and some are exceptional.

Some are available as both movies and books. Some embody the art of caring, the key philosophy of the book. They are not listed in any priority order and the list is by no means complete. Other relevant books are listed in the chapter reference lists.

Novels

Pasternak B. (1958) *Dr Zhivago*. London, Vintage Books.
Mitchell M. (1936) *Gone with the Wind*. London, Macmillan.
Dostoevsky F. (1866) *Crime and Punishment*.
Salinger JD. (1951) *The Catcher in the Rye*. San Francisco, CA, Little Brown.
Tolstoy L. (1875) *Anna Karenina*. Moscow, Russian Herald.
Tolstoy L. (1980) *War and Peace*. London, Penguin, Books.
Burge J. (2004) *(translator) Heloise and Abelard*. London, Profile Books.
Dean D. (2006) *The Madonnas of Leningrad*. London, Harper.
Ondaatje M. (1993) *The English Patient*. London New York City, Knopf Doubleday.
Tolkien JRR. (1965) *The Lord of the Rings*. London, Houghton Mifflin.
Kesey K. (1962) *One Flew over the Cuckoo's Nest*. Melbourne, Victoria, Australia, Picador.
Lawrence D. (1948) *Sons and Lovers*. London, Penguin.
Harper L. (1988) *To Kill a Mockingbird*. New York, Grand Central Publishing.
Wilde O. (2006) *Picture of Dorian Gray*. London, Norton Edition.
Sun Tzu *The Art of War*. Manhattan, Barnes and Noble.
Xenophon. (2007) *The Art of Horsemanship*, translated by Morgan M. London, JA Allen.

Diabetes Education: Art, Science and Evidence, First Edition. Edited by Trisha Dunning AM.
© 2013 by John Wiley & Sons, Ltd. Published 2013 by John Wiley & Sons, Ltd.

Alexander P (1964) *The Complete Works of William Shakespeare: Player's Edition.* London, Collins.
Higgins J. (1975) *The Eagle Has Landed.* London, Bantam Books.
Bach R. (1975) *Jonathan Livingston Seagull.* Edinburgh, Macmillan.
Stevens G. (1959) *The Diary of Anne Frank.* London, Random House.
Evans N. (1995) *The Horse Whisperer.* New York, Delacorte Press.
Lagg J. (undated) (translator) Lao Tzu *Tao Te Ching.* New York, Abrams.
Bragg M. (2003) *The Adventure of English: The Biography of a Language.* London, Hodder.

Children's books (but messages for adults too)

Williams M. (1922) *The Velveteen Rabbit.* New York Doubleday.
Ingpen R. (1986) *The Idle Bear.* Melbourne, Victoria, Australia, Lothian.
Milne AA *Winnie the Pooh.*
Lewis Carroll. (2009) *Alice in Wonderland.* London, Random House.
Sewell A. (1878) *Black Beauty.*

Poetry

Vikram S. (1999) *On Golden Gate.* London, Faber and Faber.
Pushkin A. (1977) *Eugene Onegin.* London, Penguin.
Leonard J. (1976) *Seven Centuries of English Poetry.* Oxford, Oxford University Press.
Barnstone W. (2009) *The Complete Poems of Sappho.* Boston, MA, Shambhala.
Portal J. (2004) *Chinese Love Poetry.* London, British Museum Press.
Basho. (1973) *The Narrow Road to the Deep North and Other Travels Sketches.* London, Penguin.
Everyman's Library. (1962) *Sir Gawain and the Green Knight.* London, Dent Books.
Penguin Anthology of Australian Poetry. (2009).

Personal experience

Dosa O. (2010) *Making the Rounds with Oscar.* London, Headline.
Cousin N. (1991) *Anatomy of an Illness.* New York City, Bantam Books.
Groopman G. (2007) *How Doctor's Think.* Melbourne, Victoria, Australia, Scribe.
Kaminsky L. (2010) *The Pen and the Stethoscope.* Melbourne, Victoria, Australia, Scribe.
Sanders L. (2007) *Every Patient Tells a Story.* New York, Broadway Press.

Psychology and education

Gladwell M. (2000) *The Tipping Point: How Little Things Make a Difference.* London, Abacus.
Palmer P. (1988) *The Courage to Teach: Exploring the Inner Landscape of a Teacher's Life.* San Francisco, CA, Jossey-Bass.

Bennett S, MacLean R. (2008) *Understanding Learners*. Melbourne, Victoria, Australia, Deakin University.

Jones K, Creedy D. (2008) *Health and Human Behaviour*. Oxford, Oxford University Press.

Bradshaw M, Lowenstein A (2007) *Innovative Teaching Strategies in Nursing*. Boston, MA, Jones and Bartlett.

Tubbs N. (2005) *The Philosophy of the Teacher*. Oxford, Blackwell Publishing.

Bolton R. (2009) *People Skills*. Sydney, New South Wales, Australia, Simon Schuster.

Cigman R, Davis A. (2007) *New Philosophies of Learning*. Oxford, Wiley Blackwell.

Montague R. (2006) *How We Make Decisions*. London, Plume.

Movies

Dances with Wolves	The Dead Poet's Society
Dr Zhivago	The Doctor
Finding Nemo	The Getting of Wisdom
Gone with the Wind	The Interview
Goodbye Mr Chips	The Iron Lady
Mrs Doubtfire	The Karate Kid
My Fair Lady	The King's Speech
Out of Africa	The Man in the Iron Mask
Phantom of the Opera	The Notebook
The Black Swan	The Magnificant Seven

Index

Note: Page numbers in *italics* refer to Figures; those in **bold** to Tables.